Clinical Applications of Human Neuroscience

of **Human Neuroscience**

A Laboratory Guide

Clinical Applications
of Human
Neuroscience
A Laboratory Guide

MICHAEL F. NOLAN, PhD, PT

Professor and Vice Chair
Department of Basic Sciences
Virginia Tech Carilion School of Medicine and Research Institute
Roanoke, Virginia

Professor Emeritus
Department of Pathology and Cell Biology
Morsani School of Medicine
University of South Florida
Tampa, Florida

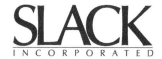

SLACK
INCORPORATED

www.Healio.com/books

ISBN: 978-1-61711-643-8

Published by: SLACK Incorporated
                  6900 Grove Road
                  Thorofare, NJ 08086 USA
                  Telephone: 856-848-1000
                  Fax: 856-848-6091
                  www.Healio.com/books

Contact SLACK Incorporated for more information about other books in this field or about the availability of our books from distributors outside the United States.

Library of Congress Cataloging-in-Publication Data
Nolan, Michael F., 1947- author.
  Clinical applications of human neuroscience : a laboratory guide / Michael F. Nolan.
    p. ; cm.
  Human neuroscience
  Includes index.
  ISBN 978-1-61711-643-8 (alk. paper)
  I. Title. II. Title: Human neuroscience.
  [DNLM: 1. Nervous System Physiological Phenomena--Laboratory Manuals. 2. Nervous System Physiological Phenomena--Problems and Exercises. 3. Neurosciences--Laboratory Manuals. 4. Neurosciences--Problems and Exercises. WL 25]
  QP360.5
  612.8'233--dc23
                                201304429

Last digit is print number: 10 9 8 7 6 5 4 3 2 1

Contents

ACKNOWLEDGMENTS

The written questions and active learning exercises included in this laboratory manual have been used, revised, reused, and re-revised many times over several years in an attempt to ensure that they are clear, instructive, meaningful, and—whenever possible—fun. Many students at many different stages in their health care careers have been involved in the development of these exercises. Most have provided feedback and suggestions along the way. My hope is that this manual will be of value to you, the current reader.

Among those who have been most helpful, I must include many classes of neurology residents, neurosurgery residents, physical therapy students, and first-year medical students whom I have had the privilege of teaching during my long career at the Morsani School of Medicine at the University of South Florida. More recently, I must acknowledge the helpful comments and recommendations from the neurosurgery residents and medical students of the Virginia Tech Carilion School of Medicine and Research Institute in Roanoke, where I am still privileged to be teaching.

It would be unthinkable to not acknowledge the support of my wonderful wife and best friend, Debby, during work not only on this book, but my previous books as well.

Finally, I take great pleasure in acknowledging John Bond, Brien Cummings, and their helpful staff at SLACK Incorporated, with whom I have worked in the past and have enjoyed working with again on this project.

About the Author

Michael F. Nolan, PhD, PT received a bachelor's degree in physical therapy from Marquette University and a PhD in anatomy (neuroanatomy) from the Medical College of Wisconsin.

Dr. Nolan is currently Professor and Vice Chair of the Department of Basic Sciences at the Virginia Tech Carilion School of Medicine and Research Institute in Roanoke, Virginia. He is also Professor Emeritus of Pathology and Cell Biology in the Morsani School of Medicine at the University of South Florida in Tampa, where he received numerous awards for teaching at both the undergraduate and graduate medical education levels, including the John M. Thompson, MD Outstanding Teacher Award in Neurosurgery.

He is the author of *Clinical Applications of Human Anatomy: A Laboratory Guide* and *Cram Session in Functional Neuroanatomy: A Handbook for Students & Clinicians*, both published by SLACK Incorporated, and *Introduction to the Neurologic Examination*.

INTRODUCTION

Students today clearly prefer learning activities that provide for active engagement, provide for some degree of independence, and make clear their applicability and value. Hands-on learning activities and opportunities that allow the student to self-monitor progress and judge success are typically high on the list of ways that students like to learn. This laboratory manual was conceived out of the desire to create learning activities that would help achieve the above-mentioned goals.

I have found over the course of my career in medical education that when students can do something as part of the learning process, they seem to retain knowledge and skills better and have more fun at the same time. For human neuroscience, learning and self-assessment activities that can be applied to the neurological examination seemed the most appropriate.

This manual is composed of 2 types of learning activities: 1) fill-in-the-blank questions that are focused on the principles and facts of neuroanatomy and neurophysiology that underpin the neurological examination and 2) group activities that demonstrate how these principles and facts are related to the particular tests and procedures that make up the neurological examination. Fill-in-the-blank questions form the bulk of the Neuroscience Review section of each chapter and are intended as a review of information previously or concurrently being learned regarding the structure, function, and organization of the nervous system. Some questions focus on anatomical or physiological facts and relationships that help explain why and how certain techniques are performed, such as why non-nociceptive tactile stimuli are required in order to activate nerve impulse transmission in the lemniscal system. Other questions are intended to revisit facts and concepts that are needed to properly interpret the elicited findings.

The group activities that compose the Application Exercises section of each chapter are designed to demonstrate how neuroanatomical and neurophysiological information is used in the design of particular clinical tests of neurological function. The application exercises are also intended to help students learn how to perform and become comfortable with the various clinical maneuvers and tests that compose the routine neurological examination. An important outcome of performing these exercises is that, as a member of a learning group, each individual has the opportunity to experience the neurological examination from the point of view of the subject (patient)—an experience that provides insight and understanding that can be gained in no other way.

The exercises in the manual are designed as active learning exercises that might complement and reinforce learning in a more traditionally structured course dealing with the clinical examination of a patient. The "group activity" approach, in which the student performs each exercise on a small number of "normal" subjects (classmates), is founded on the belief that the ability to recognize an abnormal finding on clinical examination requires a familiarity with the range of normal findings in the otherwise healthy population. This is particularly true for those who are learning about the structure and function of the nervous system for the first time.

It is my hope that the questions and exercises in this manual will help the reader acquire and solidify both knowledge and skill in evaluating the function of the nervous system.

How to Use This Manual

The exercises described in this manual are group activities, intended and designed for small numbers of students working together. Each work group should ideally consist of 4 to 6 students, preferably mixed with regard to gender, race, ethnicity, body size, and overall shape. The intent of building diversity within the work group is to permit students to gain familiarity with a wide range of normal findings. Students should dress comfortably in clothing that does not prohibit the proper performance of the exercises described.

Each student in the work group should perform each exercise on all members of the group and take a turn as subject for each of the other members. In this way, students can begin the process of gaining familiarity with the range of normal for a particular examination technique and begin to recognize differences among individuals that may affect how the test is performed or how the results are interpreted. In addition, students can begin to gain an appreciation of what it may be like to be the patient in a clinical encounter. Clearly, the greatest benefit is achieved when each student performs each exercise on all of the members of his or her group.

Although these exercises are intended to be performed during regularly scheduled laboratory sessions when faculty or preceptor assistance may be available, there is no reason why they cannot be performed or repeated outside scheduled class time. Both technical skill and the ability to reliably interpret exam results are best developed by practice and conscious reflection. There are simply no substitutes for direct experience and practice.

It is essential that you come to each scheduled laboratory session with all the diagnostic tools and other supplies that will be necessary to complete the exercises. Briefly review the exercises before each session so that you know what to bring in order to benefit from the exercises. Please be conscientious in this regard.

Finally, learning by application, particularly when it involves human subjects, can sometimes be uncomfortable or embarrassing for both the learner and the subjects, whether they are classmates or actual patients. Please view these exercises as important, necessary, and serious parts of your educational and professional development, and treat your work group partners with the respect and sensitivity you would wish them to extend to you.

SECTION I

Sensory Systems

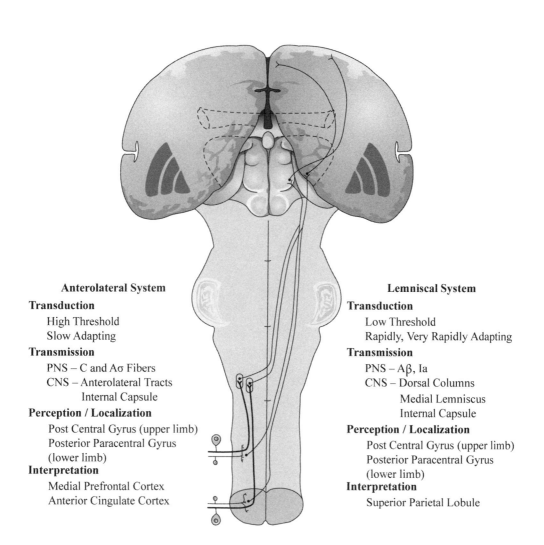

Anterolateral System

Transduction
  High Threshold
  Slow Adapting
Transmission
  PNS – C and Aσ Fibers
  CNS – Anterolateral Tracts
    Internal Capsule
Perception / Localization
  Post Central Gyrus (upper limb)
  Posterior Paracentral Gyrus
  (lower limb)
Interpretation
  Medial Prefrontal Cortex
  Anterior Cingulate Cortex

Lemniscal System

Transduction
  Low Threshold
  Rapidly, Very Rapidly Adapting
Transmission
  PNS – Aβ, Ia
  CNS – Dorsal Columns
    Medial Lemniscus
    Internal Capsule
Perception / Localization
  Post Central Gyrus (upper limb)
  Posterior Paracentral Gyrus
  (lower limb)
Interpretation
  Superior Parietal Lobule

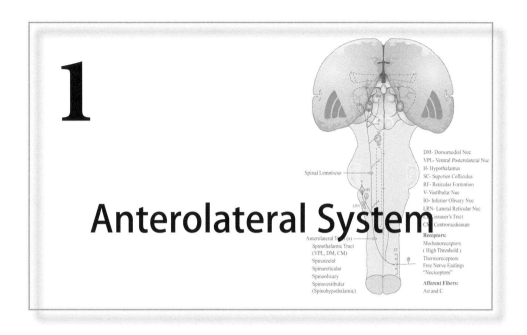

1

Anterolateral System

Spinal Lemniscus

DM- Dorsomedial Nuc
VPL- Ventral Posterolateral Nuc
H- Hypothalamus
SC- Superior Colliculus
RF- Reticular Formation
V- Vestibular Nuc
IO- Inferior Olivary Nuc
LRN- Lateral Reticular Nuc
Lissauer's Tract
CM- Centromedianum

Anterolateral Tract (s)
Spinothalamic Tract
(VPL, DM, CM)
Spinotectal
Spinoreticular
Spinoolivary
Spinovestibular
(Spinohypothalamic)

Receptors:
Mechanoreceptors
(High Threshold)
Thermoreceptors
Free Nerve Endings
"Nociceptors"

Afferent Fibers:
Aσ and C

NEUROSCIENCE REVIEW

1. **What are the characteristics of the receptors that, when activated, give rise to nerve impulse transmission in the anterolateral system?**

    a. threshold _____

    b. adapting _____

2. **What types of energy can depolarize nociceptors?**

    _____
    _____
    _____

3. **Which afferent nerve fibers transmit nerve impulses toward the central nervous system in response to activation of nociceptors? What is the conduction velocity for each fiber type?**

Fiber Type	Conduction Velocity
_____	_____
_____	_____

Nolan MF. *Clinical Applications of Human Neuroscience: A Laboratory Guide* (pp 3-7).
© 2014 SLACK Incorporated.

4. In what part of the spinal gray matter do nociceptive afferent fibers terminate?

_____

5. In which specific laminae of Rexed do nociceptive afferent fibers terminate?

_____

6. Name the region of the spinal cord where axons destined to form the anterolateral tracts decussate.

_____

7. List 2 major nuclei or regions of the brainstem that receive synaptic input from anterolateral system axons.

a. _____

b. _____

8. List 3 thalamic nuclei that receive synaptic input from anterolateral system axons.

a. _____

b. _____

c. _____

9. Cells of the ventral posterolateral nucleus project axons that terminate in the ipsilateral cerebral hemisphere. List the 2 gyri where these axons terminate and indicate the body part functionally related to each.

Gyrus	Body Part
a. _____	_____
b. _____	_____

10. In which limb of the internal capsule are these thalamocortical fibers located?

_____

11. Cells of the dorsal medial nucleus are the origin of axons that terminate in the ipsilateral cerebral hemisphere. List 2 gyri or parts of the hemisphere where these axons terminate.

a. _____

b. _____

12. **In which limb of the internal capsule are these thalamocortical fibers located?**

     _____

13. **Describe the orientation of the sensory homunculus on the primary somatosensory cortices.**

     _____

     _____

14. **Define the following terms.**

    a.   anesthesia _____

         _____

    b.   analgesia _____

         _____

    c.   hypesthesia _____

         _____

    d.   hypalgesia _____

         _____

    e.   hyperalgesia _____

         _____

    f.   allodynia _____

         _____

    g.   paresthesia _____

         _____

    h.   dysesthesia _____

         _____

    i.   nociceptor _____

         _____

Application Exercises

1.   On several lab partners, identify the area of skin innervated by each of the following pre-plexus spinal nerves:

   a.   upper limb—C5, C6, C7, C8, T1

   b.   trunk—T4, T10

   c.   lower limb—L2, L3, L4, L5, S1

2.   With a skin pencil, mark the autonomous zone for each of the above-listed pre-plexus spinal nerves.

3.   On several lab partners, identify the area of skin innervated by each of the following post-plexus peripheral nerves.

Upper Limb

   a.   median   _____

   b.   ulnar   _____

   c.   radial   _____

   d.   axillary   _____

   e.   musculocutaneous   _____

   f.   medial antebrachial cutaneous   _____

   g.   medial brachial cutaneous   _____

Lower Limb

   a.   lateral femoral cutaneous   _____

   b.   obturator   _____

   c.   deep peroneal (fibular)   _____

   d.   superficial peroneal (fibular)   _____

   e.   saphenous   _____

   f.   sural   _____

4.   With a skin pencil, mark the autonomous zone for each of the above-listed post-plexus peripheral nerves.

5. On several lab partners, demonstrate and describe a method for evaluating the anterolateral system in a patient with a suspected lesion in the posterior limb of the internal capsule.

6. On several lab partners, demonstrate and describe a method for evaluating the anterolateral system in a patient with a suspected lesion involving the radial nerve.

7. On several lab partners, demonstrate and describe a method for evaluating the anterolateral system in a patient with a suspected distal peripheral neuropathy such as that found in a patient with diabetes mellitus.

8. Which peripheral nervous system structure is most likely involved in a patient with absent pin prick sensation on the skin of the palmar surface of the left long finger? On which side is the lesion?

Structure Involved   Side of Lesion

_____   _____

9. What peripheral nervous system structure is most likely involved in a patient with absent thermal sensation on the skin of the lateral surface of the right thigh? On which side is the lesion?

Structure Involved   Side of Lesion

_____   _____

10. Which limb(s) is(are) most likely to be affected in a patient with sensory impairment resulting from damage to Lissauer's tract on the left side extending from C5–T1? Which side of the body is affected?

Limb(s) Affected   Side Affected

_____   _____

_____   _____

11. Which limb of the internal capsule is most likely involved in a patient with increased threshold to pin prick stimulation of the left upper and lower limbs? On which side is the lesion?

Part of Internal Capsule   Side of the Lesion

_____   _____

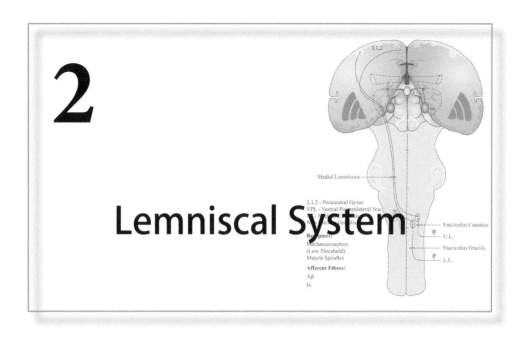

2

Lemniscal System

Medial Lemniscus

3,1,2 - Postcentral Gyrus
VPL - Ventral Posterolateral Nuc.
N.C. - Nucleus Cuneatus
N.G. - Nucleus Gracilis

Receptors:
Mechanoreceptors
(Low Threshold)
Muscle Spindles

Afferent Fibers:
Aβ
Ia

Fasciculus Cuneatus

U.L.

Fasciculus Gracilis

L.L.

NEUROSCIENCE REVIEW

1. **What are the characteristics of the receptors that, when activated, give rise to nerve impulse transmission in the lemniscal system?**

   a. threshold _____

   b. adapting _____

2. **Which receptor is involved in the perception of light tactile stimuli?**

   _____

3. **Which receptor is primarily involved in the perception of joint position and movement?**

   _____

Nolan MF. *Clinical Applications of Human Neuroscience:*
A Laboratory Guide (pp 9-15).
© 2014 SLACK Incorporated.

4. Which afferent nerve fiber transmits nerve impulses toward the central nervous system in response to activation of receptors involved in the perception of light tactile stimuli, and what is its conduction velocity?

Fiber Type	Conduction Velocity
_____	_____

5. Which afferent nerve fiber transmits nerve impulses toward the central nervous system in response to activation of receptors involved in the perception of joint position and movement, and what is its conduction velocity?

Fiber Type	Conduction Velocity
_____	_____
_____	_____

6. In which funiculus of the spinal cord are the central processes of these non-nociceptive afferent cells located?

_____

7. Name the 2 fasciculi in the spinal cord that are formed by the central processes of non-nociceptive afferent fibers and indicate which limb is associated with each.

Fasciculus	Limb
a. _____	_____
b. _____	_____

8. Describe the somatotopic organization of the fibers of the dorsal funiculus.

_____

_____

9. List the nuclei where these fibers terminate and indicate the part of the body functionally related to each.

Nucleus	Body Part
_____	_____
_____	_____

10. At what level of the brainstem do the axons of the above 2 nuclei cross the midline? (Be as specific as you can.)

    _____

    _____

11. Which fiber tract is formed by these axons after they cross the midline?

    _____

12. What is the somatotopic organization of this pathway at the level of the:

    a. inferior olivary nucleus _____

    b. mid pons _____

    c. mid midbrain_____

13. Name the thalamic nucleus where the fibers of the medial lemniscus terminate.

    _____

14. Describe the somatotopic organization of the cells of this thalamic nucleus.

    _____

15. Cells of the ventral posterolateral nucleus project axons that terminate in the ipsilateral cerebral hemisphere. List the 2 gyri where these axons terminate and indicate the body part functionally related to each.

Gyrus	Body Part
a. _____	_____
b. _____	_____

16. In which limb of the internal capsule are these thalamocortical fibers located?

_____

17. Describe the orientation of the sensory homunculus on the primary somatosensory cortices.

_____

18. Which 2 functions of a sensory system occur as a result of activating the primary somatosensory cortex?

a. _____

b. _____

19. Cells of the primary somatosensory cortex project axons toward 2 other regions of the cerebral cortex. What are these other cortical areas and what (briefly) are their functions?

Cortical Area   Function

a. _____   _____

b. _____   _____

20. Define the following terms.

a. hypesthesia _____

_____

b. hyperesthesia _____

_____

c. thigmesthesia _____

_____

d. pallesthesia _____

_____

e. proprioception _____

_____

f.   kinesthesia _____

_____

g.   topesthesia _____

_____

APPLICATION EXERCISES

1.   **On several lab partners, identify the area of skin innervated by each of the following pre-plexus spinal nerves:**

   a.   upper limb—C5, C6, C7, C8, T1

   b.   trunk—T4, T10

   c.   lower limb—L2, L3, L4, L5, S1

2.   **With a skin pencil, mark the autonomous zone for each of the above-listed pre-plexus spinal nerves.**

3.   **On several lab partners, identify the area of skin innervated by each of the following peripheral nerves.**

Upper Limb

   a.   median   _____

   b.   ulnar   _____

   c.   radial   _____

   d.   axillary   _____

   e.   musculocutaneous   _____

   f.   medial antebrachial cutaneous   _____

   g.   medial brachial cutaneous   _____

Lower Limb

   a.   lateral femoral cutaneous   _____

   b.   obturator   _____

   c.   deep peroneal (fibular)   _____

   d.   superficial peroneal (fibular)   _____

e.   saphenous   _____

f.   sural   _____

4.   With a skin pencil, mark the autonomous zone for each of the above-listed post-plexus peripheral nerves.

5.   On several lab partners, demonstrate and describe a method for evaluating light touch perception in the upper and lower limbs.

6.   Describe the findings you would expect on testing light touch sensation in a patient with a suspected lesion in the posterior limb of the internal capsule on the right side.

_____

_____

7.   On several lab partners, demonstrate and describe a method for evaluating tactile localization in the upper and lower limbs.

8.   Describe the findings you would expect on testing light touch sensation in a patient with a suspected lesion in the radial nerve on the left side.

_____

_____

9.   Which tuning fork should be used for testing vibratory sense?

_____

10.   On several lab partners, demonstrate and describe a method for evaluating vibratory sense in the upper and lower limbs.

11.   Describe the findings you might expect on testing vibratory sense in a patient with a suspected distal peripheral neuropathy such as might be found in a patient with diabetes mellitus.

_____

_____

12.   On several lab partners, demonstrate and describe a method for evaluating position sense in the upper and lower limbs.

13. Describe the findings you might expect on testing position sense in a patient with a suspected distal peripheral neuropathy such as that found in a patient with diabetes mellitus.

    _____

    _____

14. On several lab partners, demonstrate and describe a method for evaluating station using the Romberg test.

15. Describe the findings you would observe in a patient in whom the Romberg test is positive.

    _____

    _____

16. Where might a lesion be located in a patient who demonstrates a positive Romberg test?

    _____

17. Which spinal pathway is most likely involved in a patient with impaired vibratory sensation in the right foot? On which side of the spinal cord is the lesion?

    Spinal Pathway   **Side of Lesion**

    _____   _____

18. Which thalamic nucleus is most likely involved in a patient with increased threshold to light touch stimuli in the left upper and lower limbs? On which side of the brain is the lesion?

    Thalamic Nucleus   **Side of Lesion**

    _____   _____

19. An imaging study in a patient with impaired vibratory sense and increased threshold to non-nociceptive cutaneous stimuli in the left upper and lower limbs reveals a focal abnormality in the caudal pons. What neural structure is most likely involved and on which side?

    Neural Structure   **Side of Lesion**

    _____   _____

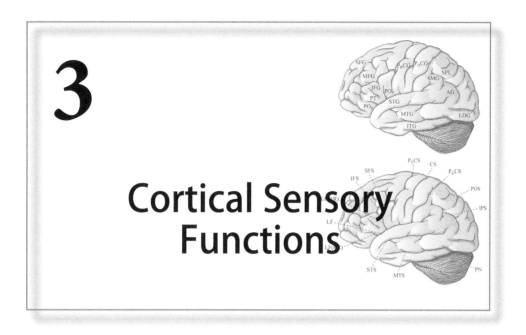

3

Cortical Sensory Functions

NEUROSCIENCE REVIEW

1. Which gyrus and Brodmann areas are referred to as primary somatosensory cortex for the upper limb?

Gyrus   **Brodmann Areas**

_____   _____

2. Which cortical and Brodmann areas are referred to as somatosensory association areas for the upper limb?

Cortical Area   **Brodmann Areas**

_____   _____

3. Which artery supplies blood to the primary somatosensory cortex for the upper limb?

_____

4. Which frequency tuning fork is used to evaluate vibratory sense?

_____

Nolan MF. *Clinical Applications of Human Neuroscience: A Laboratory Guide* (pp 17-19). © 2014 SLACK Incorporated.

5.   **Which digits in the upper and lower limbs are commonly used to evaluate position sense?**

a.   upper limb _____

b.   lower limb _____

6.   **Define the following terms.**

a.   proprioception (position sense) _____

_____

b.   graphesthesia (traced figure identification) _____

_____

c.   stereognosia (object identification) _____

_____

d.   somatosensory neglect _____

_____

e.   tactile agnosia _____

_____

f.   extinction to double simultaneous stimulation _____

_____

g.   kinesthesia _____

_____

APPLICATION EXERCISES

1.   **On several lab partners, demonstrate and describe a method for evaluating position sense in the upper and lower limbs.**

2.   **How many trials (position changes) should you perform to obtain a reliable evaluation?**

_____

3.   **Approximately how many degrees of arc should you move a joint through when evaluating position sense?**

_____

4.   On several lab partners, demonstrate and describe a method for evaluating graphesthesia (traced figure identification).

5.   On several lab partners, demonstrate and describe a method for evaluating stereognosia (object identification).

6.   On several lab partners, demonstrate and describe a method for evaluating somatosensory extinction (extinction to double simultaneous stimulation).

7.   In a patient with a lesion in the right parietal lobe, which side of the body will demonstrate somatosensory extinction?

SECTION II

Motor Systems

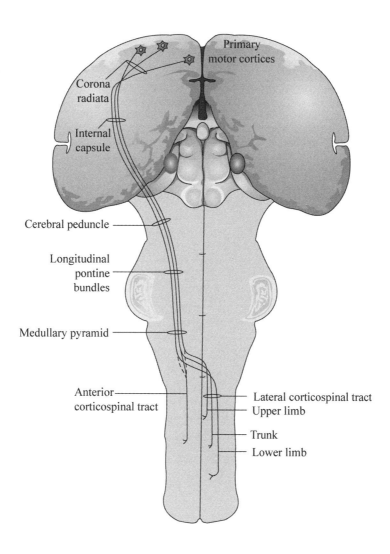

Primary motor cortices

Corona radiata

Internal capsule

Cerebral peduncle

Longitudinal pontine bundles

Medullary pyramid

Anterior corticospinal tract

Lateral corticospinal tract
Upper limb

Trunk

Lower limb

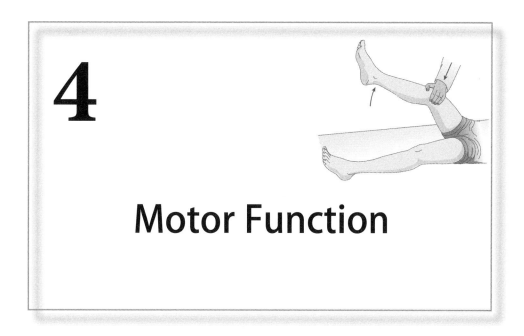

4

Motor Function

Neuroscience Review

1. Indicate the peripheral nerve being tested when you evaluate the strength of each of the following movements.

Upper Limb		**Peripheral Nerve**
a.	shoulder abduction	_____
b.	elbow flexion	_____
c.	elbow extension	_____
d.	wrist extension	_____
e.	wrist flexion	_____
f.	finger extension	_____
g.	finger flexion (grip strength)	_____
h.	finger abduction	_____
i.	finger adduction	_____

Nolan MF. *Clinical Applications of Human Neuroscience:*
A Laboratory Guide (pp 23-30).
© 2014 SLACK Incorporated.

Lower Limb   ## Peripheral Nerve

a.   hip flexion

b.   hip adduction   _____

c.   hip abduction   _____

d.   hip extension   _____

e.   knee extension   _____

f.   knee flexion   _____

g.   ankle dorsiflexion   _____

h.   ankle plantar flexion   _____

i.   toe extension   _____

2.   **Indicate the spinal segments being tested when you evaluate the strength of each of the following movements.**

Upper Limb   ## Spinal Segments

a.   shoulder abduction   _____

b.   elbow flexion   _____

c.   elbow extension   _____

d.   wrist extension   _____

e.   wrist flexion   _____

f.   finger extension   _____

g.   finger flexion (grip strength)   _____

h.   finger abduction   _____

i.   finger adduction   _____

Lower Limb   ## Spinal Segments

a.   hip flexion   _____

b.   hip adduction   _____

c.   hip abduction   _____

d.   hip extension   _____

e.   knee extension   _____

f.   knee flexion   _____

g.   ankle dorsiflexion   _____

h.   ankle plantar flexion   _____

i.   toe extension   _____

3.   **Which lobes of the brain contain corticospinal tract cell bodies?**

_____

_____

4.   **Which lobe(s) of the brain contain(s) cortical upper motor neurons that influence lower motor neurons that innervate muscles of the:**

a.   upper limbs _____

b.   lower limbs _____

5.   **Which gyrus(gyri) contain(s) cortical upper motor neurons that influence lower motor neurons that innervate muscles of the:**

a.   upper limbs _____

b.   lower limbs _____

6.   **In which white matter structure of the brain are corticospinal axons located at the level of the:**

a.   thalamus _____

b.   midbrain _____

c.   pons _____

d.   medulla oblongata _____

7.   **What is the name of the white matter structure where corticospinal fibers decussate (cross the midline)?**

_____

8.   **Which limb is influenced by corticospinal fibers that decussate in the:**

a.   rostral part of the pyramidal decussation _____

b.   caudal part of the pyramidal decussation _____

9.   **What percentage of corticospinal fibers typically decussates in the pyramidal decussation?**

_____

10. **Which descending spinal cord pathway is formed by corticospinal fibers that:**

    a.   decussate in the pyramidal decussation _____

    b.   do not decussate in the pyramidal decussation _____

11. **What percentage of fibers of the lateral corticospinal tract terminates at:**

    a.   upper limb segments (C5–T1)_____

    b.   lower limb segments (L2–S2) _____

    c.   non-limb segments _____

12. **In segments of the spinal cord that contain lower motor neurons that innervate the limbs, which muscle groups are innervated by lower motor neurons primarily located in the:**

Muscle Groups

    a.   medial part of the ventral horn   _____

    b.   intermediate part of the ventral horn _____

    c.   lateral part of the ventral horn   _____

13. **Define the performance criteria/characteristics for each of the following muscle strength grades.**

    a.   normal (5/5) _____

          _____

    b.   good (4/5) _____

          _____

    c.   fair (3/5) _____

          _____

    d.   poor (2/5) _____

          _____

    e.   trace (1/5) _____

          _____

    f.   zero (0/5) _____

          _____

14. Define the following terms.

a. motor unit _____

_____

b. disuse atrophy _____

_____

c. denervation atrophy_____

_____

d. hypertrophy _____

_____

e. paresis_____

_____

f. hemiparesis _____

_____

g. paralysis _____

_____

h. pronator drift_____

_____

i. fibrillation _____

_____

j. fasciculation _____

_____

k. paraplegia_____

_____

l. quadriplegia _____

_____

m. wrist drop_____

_____

n. foot drop _____

_____

o. claw hand _____

_____

p. Erb's palsy _____

_____

q. Klumpke's palsy _____

_____

APPLICATION EXERCISES

1. Inspect and compare the 2 upper limbs and the 2 lower limbs. Focus on symmetry, specifically regarding muscle bulk and contour. Describe and characterize any observed asymmetry or side-to-side differences in bulk and contour.

2. Is observed asymmetry necessarily a sign of abnormality or pathology?

_____

3. If not, how much asymmetry might be seen in the normal population and how might you explain the presence of visible asymmetry between muscles or muscle groups?

_____

_____

4. On several lab partners, demonstrate and describe how to measure strength of each of the following movements and assign an appropriate strength grade.

Upper Limb   Strength Grade

a. shoulder abduction   _____

b. elbow flexion   _____

c. elbow extension   _____

d. wrist extension   _____

e. wrist flexion   _____

f. finger extension   _____

g. finger flexion (grip strength)   _____

h. finger abduction   _____

i. finger adduction   _____

Lower Limb   ## Strength Grade

a. hip flexion   _____

b. hip adduction   _____

c. hip abduction   _____

d. hip extension   _____

e. knee extension   _____

f. knee flexion   _____

g. ankle dorsiflexion   _____

h. ankle plantar flexion   _____

i. toe extension   _____

5. **What are the likely locations of lesions that result in denervation atrophy?**

_____

_____

6. **Which peripheral nervous system structure is most likely involved in a patient with 0/5 strength of ankle dorsiflexion and 0/5 strength of great toe extension on the right side? Which side is involved?**

Structure Involved   ### Side of Lesion

_____   _____

7. **Which peripheral nervous system structure is most likely involved in a patient with 3/5 strength of elbow flexion and 3/5 strength of shoulder abduction on the left side? Which side is involved?**

Structure Involved   ### Side of Lesion

_____   _____

8. **Which peripheral nervous system structure is most likely involved in a patient with 0/5 strength of finger abduction, finger adduction, and wrist flexion with ulnar deviation on the right side? Which side is involved?**

Structure Involved   ### Side of Lesion

_____   _____

9. Which peripheral nervous system structure is most likely involved in a patient with 2/5 strength of knee extension and 3/5 strength of hip adduction on the left side? Which side is involved?

Structure Involved   **Side of Lesion**

_____   _____

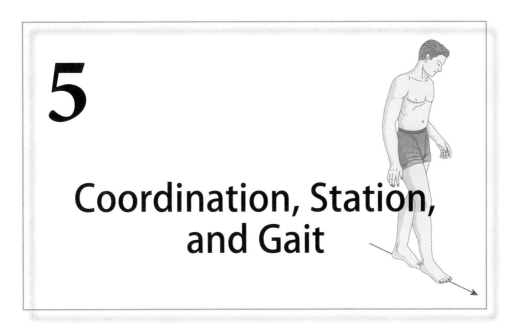

5

Coordination, Station, and Gait

NEUROSCIENCE REVIEW

1. **List the 3 gross anatomical parts of the cerebellum.**

    a. _____

    b. _____

    c. _____

2. **List the 3 developmental (embryological) components of the cerebellum.**

    a. _____

    b. _____

    c. _____

3. **List the 3 functional regions of the cerebellar cortex.**

    a. _____

    b. _____

    c. _____

Nolan MF. *Clinical Applications of Human Neuroscience:*
A Laboratory Guide (pp 31-37).
© 2014 SLACK Incorporated.

4.　Name the fissure that separates the anterior lobe from the posterior lobe.

　　　_____

5.　Name the fissure that separates the posterior lobe from the flocculonodular lobe.

　　　_____

6.　Name the 3 major cerebellar peduncles and the region of the brainstem with which each is anatomically associated.

	Cerebellar Peduncle	Associated Brainstem Region
a.	_____	_____
b.	_____	_____
c.	_____	_____

7.　Name the 3 layers of the cerebellar cortex.

　　a.　_____

　　b.　_____

　　c.　_____

8.　Name the 2 cells with cell bodies located in the molecular layer.

　　a.　_____

　　b.　_____

9.　Name the 2 cells with cell bodies located in the granular layer.

　　a.　_____

　　b.　_____

10. List the major cerebellar afferent and efferent tracts located in each of the cerebellar peduncles.

		Afferent Tract	**Efferent Tract**
a.	superior cerebellar peduncle	_____	_____
		_____	_____
			_____
b.	middle cerebellar peduncle	_____	
c.	inferior cerebellar peduncle	_____	
		_____	
		_____	
d.	juxtarestiform body	_____	_____

11. What nucleus is the origin of climbing fibers?

    _____

12. Name 2 nuclei in the spinal cord that are the origin of mossy fibers.

    a. _____

    b. _____

13. Name 2 nuclei in the medulla oblongata that are the origin of mossy fibers.

    a. _____

    b. _____

14. In what layer of the cerebellar cortex are glomeruli located?

    _____

15. Which cell is the "output" cell of the cerebellar cortex?

    _____

16. **What is the neurotransmitter synthesized and used by this cell?**

_____

17. **Name the cerebellar deep nuclei from medial to lateral and indicate the functional region(s) of the cerebellar cortex with which it is related.**

Nucleus	Functional Cortical Region(s)
_____	_____
_____	_____
_____	_____
_____	_____

18. **List the cerebellar deep nuclei from medial to lateral and indicate the main nucleus to which each projects.**

Nucleus	Nuclear Target
_____	_____
_____	_____
_____	_____
_____	_____

19. **Define the following terms.**

a. ataxia of gait _____

_____

b. truncal ataxia _____

_____

c. metric movements _____

_____

d. dysmetria _____

_____

e. diadochokinetic movements _____

_____

f. dysdiadochokinesia _____

_____

g. dysarthria _____

_____

h. intention (kinetic) tremor _____

_____

i. titubation _____

_____

j. check and rebound _____

_____

k. astasia _____

_____

l. astasia-abasia _____

_____

m. abnormal gait patterns

spastic gait _____

_____

antalgic gait _____

_____

hemiparetic gait _____

_____

steppage gait _____

_____

festinating gait _____

_____

APPLICATION EXERCISES

1. **On several lab partners, demonstrate and describe a method for evaluating coordination (metric movements) in the upper and lower limbs.**

2. Describe the findings you might expect from those who demonstrated dysmetria of the upper limb and of the lower limb.

a. upper limb _____

_____

b. lower limb _____

_____

3. On several lab partners, demonstrate and describe a method for evaluating coordination (diadochokinetic movements) in the upper and lower limbs.

4. Describe the findings you might expect from those who demonstrated dysdiadochokinesia of the upper limb and of the lower limb.

a. upper limb _____

_____

b. lower limb _____

_____

5. On several lab partners, demonstrate and describe a method for evaluating station using the Romberg test.

6. Describe your observations in a patient in whom the Romberg test is positive.

_____

_____

7. Where might a lesion be located in a patient who demonstrates a positive Romberg test?

_____

8. On several lab partners, demonstrate and describe a method for evaluating gait.

9. List and describe several specific components of gait on which you might focus during an evaluation of gait.

_____

_____

10. Describe the characteristics of a hemiparetic gait.

11. Describe the features of the gait of a patient with unilateral foot drop.

12. Describe the features of the gait of a patient with a destructive lesion involving the cerebellar vermis.

13. Describe the features of the gait of a patient with Parkinson's disease.

14. Describe the features of the gait of a patient with Huntington's disease.

15. Describe the features of the gait of a patient with tabes dorsalis (sensory ataxia).

16. A 27-year-old man presents with the sudden onset of difficulty walking. On examination, he demonstrates impaired performance on finger-to-nose testing and heel-to-shin testing on the right side. An imaging study reveals a tumor mass in the cerebellum. On which side is the tumor mass most likely located?

17. Lesions of the cerebellar hemisphere are sometimes associated with hypotonia. Which hemisphere of the cerebellum is most likely to be affected in a patient who demonstrates hypotonia in the left upper and lower limbs?

SECTION III

Reflexes

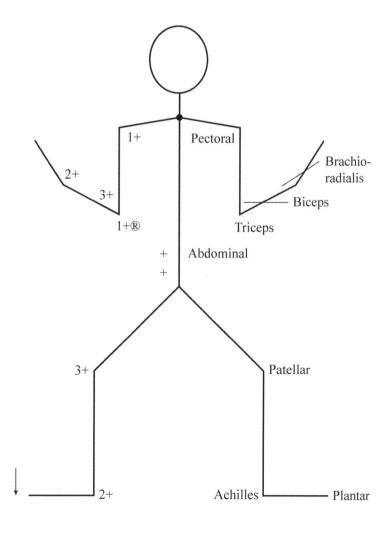

1+

Pectoral

Brachio-
radialis

2+

3+

Biceps

1+®

Triceps

+
+

Abdominal

3+

Patellar

2+

Achilles

Plantar

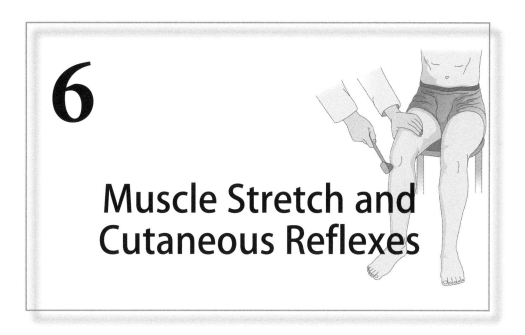

6

Muscle Stretch and Cutaneous Reflexes

NEUROSCIENCE REVIEW

1. Name the 2 muscle-related receptors that play a role in mediating muscle tone.

   a. _____

   b. _____

2. Which of these receptors is activated when eliciting a muscle stretch reflex?

   _____

3. What is the adequate stimulus for activating a muscle spindle?

   _____

4. Name the 2 types of afferent endings that are associated with the muscle spindle and indicate the afferent nerve fiber type associated with each.

Afferent Ending	Afferent Fiber Type
a. _____	_____
b. _____	_____

Nolan MF. *Clinical Applications of Human Neuroscience: A Laboratory Guide* (pp 41-47).

5.   What is the conduction velocity for each of these 2 afferent nerve fibers?

     Afferent Fiber Type   **Conduction Velocity**

     a.   _____   _____

     b.   _____   _____

6.   What is the physiological effect of activating muscle spindles on efferent (motor) cells in the central nervous system?

     _____

7.   Name the nerve cell that provides motor innervation to the muscle spindle and indicate the conduction velocity of the axon of that cell.

     Motor Cell Type   **Conduction Velocity**

     _____   _____

8.   What is the adequate stimulus for the Golgi tendon organ?

     _____

9.   Which fiber type is associated with the Golgi tendon organ and what is the conduction velocity for this afferent nerve fiber?

     Afferent Fiber Type   **Conduction Velocity**

     _____   _____

10. What is the physiological effect of activating Golgi tendon organs on efferent (motor) cells in the central nervous system?

     _____

11. List the peripheral nerves that mediate each of the following muscle stretch reflexes.

     a.   biceps reflex _____

     b.   triceps reflex _____

     c.   brachioradialis reflex _____

     d.   finger flexor reflex _____

     e.   quadriceps reflex _____

     f.   Achilles reflex _____

12. **List the spinal segments that mediate each of the following reflexes.**

    a. biceps reflex _____

    b. triceps reflex _____

    c. brachioradialis reflex _____

    d. finger flexor reflex _____

    e. quadriceps reflex _____

    f. Achilles reflex _____

13. **Define each of the following reflex grades.**

    a. 0/5 _____

    _____

    b. 1/5 _____

    _____

    c. 2/5 _____

    _____

    d. 3/5 _____

    _____

    e. 4/5 _____

    _____

    f. 5/5 _____

    _____

14. **List 3 features that characterize and distinguish spasticity from rigidity.**

    a. spasticity

        1. _____
        2. _____
        3. _____

    b. rigidity

        1. _____
        2. _____
        3. _____

15. Several muscle stretch reflexes are "suppressed" in the neurologically intact indi-
    vidual and become manifest with certain types of central nervous system injuries.
    List 2 of these normally suppressed reflexes.

    a. _____

    b. _____

16. What is the adequate stimulus for eliciting the plantar reflex?

    _____

17. What is the normal response when eliciting the plantar reflex?

    _____

18. What is the term used to refer to an abnormal plantar reflex?

    _____

19. Is an abnormal plantar reflex a sign of an upper or lower motor neuron injury?

    _____

20. Define the following terms.

    a. normal muscle tone _____

    _____

    b. atonia, hypotonia, hypertonia _____

    _____

    c. spasticity _____

    _____

    d. clonus _____

    _____

    e. reflex spread _____

    _____

    f. withdrawal reflex _____

    _____

    g. placing reaction _____

    _____

h.   lead pipe rigidity _____

_____

i.   cogwheel rigidity _____

_____

j.   rest tremor _____

_____

k.   dystonia _____

_____

l.   tics _____

_____

m.   myoclonus _____

_____

n.   athetosis _____

_____

o.   chorea _____

_____

p.   ballismus (hemiballismus) _____

_____

q.   asterixis _____

_____

r.   blepharospasm _____

_____

APPLICATION EXERCISES

1.   **On several lab partners, demonstrate and describe a method for eliciting the static component of the tonic stretch reflex.**

2.   **On several lab partners, demonstrate and describe a method for eliciting the dynamic component of the tonic stretch reflex.**

3. List the 4 observable response variables for the phasic component of the muscle stretch reflex.

    a. _____

    b. _____

    c. _____

    d. _____

4. On several lab partners, demonstrate and describe a method for evaluating muscle tone in the upper and lower limbs.

5. On several lab partners, demonstrate and describe a method for evaluating clonus in the lower limb.

6. On several lab partners, demonstrate and describe a method for eliciting each of the following muscle stretch (deep tendon) reflexes and assign an appropriate grade.

    a. biceps reflex _____

    b. triceps reflex _____

    c. brachioradialis reflex _____

    d. finger flexor reflex _____

    e. quadriceps reflex _____

    f. Achilles reflex _____

7. On several lab partners, demonstrate and describe a method for eliciting the plantar reflex.

8. Which muscle stretch reflex is most likely to be affected in a patient with a lesion involving the C7 spinal nerve on the right side? On which side would the reflex be affected?

           Reflex Affected   **Side Affected**

        _____   _____

9. Which muscle stretch reflex is most likely to be affected in a patient with a lesion involving the femoral nerve on the left side? On which side would the reflex be affected?

           Reflex Affected   **Side Affected**

        _____   _____

10. On several lab partners, demonstrate and describe a method for eliciting the abdominal reflex.

11. On several lab partners, demonstrate and describe a method for eliciting the Hoffman reflex.

SECTION IV

Cranial Nerves

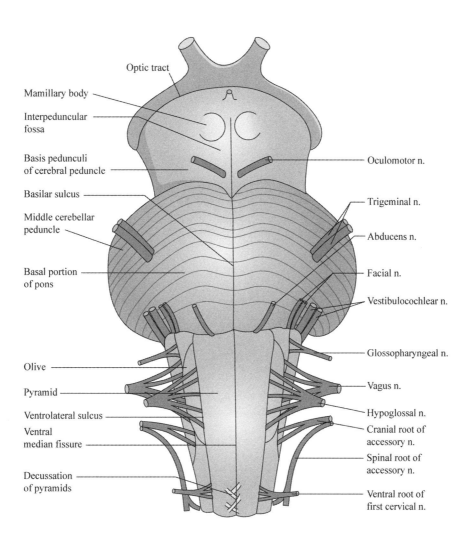

Optic tract

Mamillary body

Interpeduncular fossa

Basis pedunculi of cerebral peduncle

Basilar sulcus

Middle cerebellar peduncle

Basal portion of pons

Olive

Pyramid

Ventrolateral sulcus

Ventral median fissure

Decussation of pyramids

Oculomotor n.

Trigeminal n.

Abducens n.

Facial n.

Vestibulocochlear n.

Glossopharyngeal n.

Vagus n.

Hypoglossal n.

Cranial root of accessory n.

Spinal root of accessory n.

Ventral root of first cervical n.

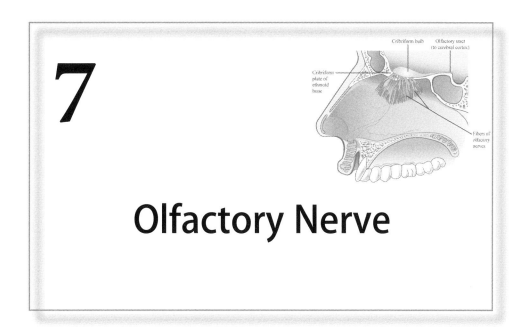

7

Olfactory Nerve

NEUROSCIENCE REVIEW

1. List the 4 cell types found in the olfactory epithelium.

    a. _____

    b. _____

    c. _____

    d. _____

2. Which of the above-listed cells is associated with a cellular process that forms the olfactory fila?

    _____

3. How do the olfactory fila gain access to the intracranial compartment?

    _____

Nolan MF. *Clinical Applications of Human Neuroscience:*
A Laboratory Guide (pp 51-53).
© 2014 SLACK Incorporated.

4.   Name the gross neural structure where the axons of the olfactory fila terminate.

_____

5.   Name the cells in the above-named structure that give rise to the axons of the olfactory tract.

_____

6.   What is the affect (excitation/inhibition) of activating cells of the anterior olfactory nucleus?

_____

7.   List 3 major targets of axons of the lateral olfactory stria.

a.   _____

b.   _____

c.   _____

8.   List 1 major synaptic target of the axons of the medial olfactory stria.

a.   _____

9.   List several odorants that might be used to evaluate olfactory function.

_____

10.   Briefly explain why you do not use irritant substances (volatile hydrocarbons such as ammonia) to test olfactory function.

_____

_____

11.   Define the following term.

a.   anosmia _____

_____

APPLICATION EXERCISES

1. On several lab partners, inspect the nares (note the position of the nasal septum and look for obstructions).

2. On several lab partners, demonstrate and describe a method for evaluating olfactory function. (Be sure to evaluate each side separately.)

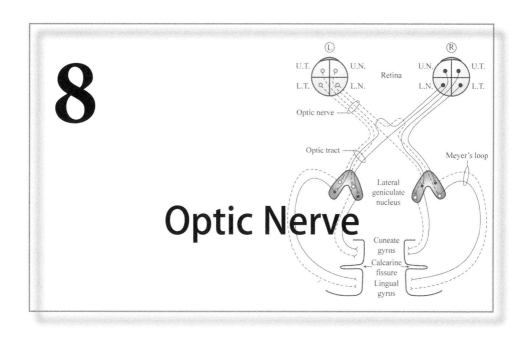

8

Optic Nerve

NEUROSCIENCE REVIEW

1. Describe the relationship between visual fields and retinal quadrants.

    _____

    _____

2. Indicate the extent of vision (in degrees of arc) in each of the 4 directions indicated below with the eye maintained in the position of primary gaze.

    a. superiorly _____

    b. medially _____

    c. inferiorly _____

    d. laterally _____

3. Describe the location and size (in degrees of arc) of the binocular visual field of an individual with both eyes viewing and in the position of primary gaze.

    _____

    _____

Nolan MF. *Clinical Applications of Human Neuroscience: A Laboratory Guide* (pp 55-62).
© 2014 SLACK Incorporated.

4. Describe the location and size (in degrees of arc) of the monocular visual fields for each eye of an individual with both eyes viewing and in the position of primary gaze.

    _____

5. Which retinal quadrants from which eye are represented in the right optic nerve?

    Retinal Quadrant   **Eye**

    _____   _____

    _____   _____

    _____   _____

    _____   _____

6. Which retinal quadrants from which eye are represented in the right optic tract?

    Retinal Quadrant   **Eye**

    _____   _____

    _____   _____

    _____   _____

    _____   _____

7. In which part of the optic chiasm will you find the decussating fibers from the macular part of each retina?

    _____

8. What percentage of the axons of the optic nerve decussates (crosses) in the optic chiasm?

    _____

9. Which retinal quadrant is represented by the axons that form Wilbrand's knee?

    _____

10. Which retinal quadrants are the origin of axons that synapse in the lateral part of the lateral geniculate nucleus on the right side?

    a. right eye _____

    b. left eye _____

11. Which retinal quadrants are the origin of axons that synapse in the medial part of the lateral geniculate nucleus on the left side?

   a.   right eye _____

   b.   left eye _____

12. Which part of the lateral geniculate nucleus is the origin of axons that course through Meyer's loop?

   _____

13. Name the gyrus of the occipital lobe that receives synaptic input from cells in each of the following:

   ## Lateral Geniculate Nucleus   Gyrus

   a.   lateral part   _____

   b.   medial part   _____

14. What part of the visual field projects visual information to the:

   a.   anterior part of the calcarine cortex _____

   b.   occipital pole _____

15. Which artery supplies the primary visual cortex?

   _____

16. Which Brodmann areas are considered visual association cortices?

   _____

17. Name the visual field defect associated with lesions affecting each of the following parts of the visual pathway (assume a complete lesion).

   a.   right optic nerve _____

   b.   left optic tract _____

   c.   optic chiasm_____

   d.   right lateral geniculate _____

   e.   left Meyer's loop _____

18. What type of vision is measured using a Snellen chart?

　　　_____

19. What type of vision is measured using a Rosenbaum card?

　　　_____

20. Where are the cell bodies of the 2 nerve cells that mediate pupillary constriction?

Preganglionic Cell　　　　**Postganglionic Cell**

　_____　　　　_____

21. Where are the cell bodies of the 2 nerve cells that mediate pupillary dilatation?

Preganglionic Cell　　　　**Postganglionic Cell**

　_____　　　　_____

22. Which nerve serves as the afferent limb of the pupillary light reflex?

　　　_____

23. Which nerve serves as the efferent limb of the pupillary light reflex?

　　　_____

24. Describe the response referred to as the direct light reflex.

　　　_____

25. Describe the response referred to as the indirect (consensual) light reflex.

　　　_____

26. List the 3 components of the accommodation response.

　　　a.　_____

　　　b.　_____

　　　c.　_____

27. What is the likely location of a lesion in a patient with a relative afferent pupillary defect on the right side?

　　　_____

28.   Define the following terms.

a.   macular vision _____

_____

b.   peripheral vision _____

_____

c.   temporal crescent _____

_____

d.   occipital pole _____

_____

e.   Meyer's loop _____

_____

f.   macular sparring _____

_____

g.   anopsia (anopia) _____

_____

h.   blind spot _____

_____

i.   hemianopsia _____

_____

j.   quadrantanopsia _____

_____

k.   homonymous _____

_____

l.   heteronymous _____

_____

m.   scotoma _____

_____

n.   positive scotoma _____

_____

o.   negative scotoma _____

_____

p.   amaurosis fugax _____

_____

q.   myopia _____

_____

r.   hyperopia _____

_____

s.   amblyopia _____

_____

t.   diplopia _____

_____

u.   miosis _____

_____

v.   mydriasis _____

_____

w.   anisocoria _____

_____

x.   iridoplegia _____

_____

y.   cycloplegia _____

_____

z.   hippus _____

_____

aa.   presbyopia _____

_____

ab.   relative afferent pupillary defect _____

_____

ac.   light-near dissociation _____

_____

ad. Marcus-Gunn pupil _____

_____

ae. Adie's pupil _____

_____

APPLICATION EXERCISES

1. **On several lab partners, demonstrate and describe a method for evaluating visual fields.**

2. **On several lab partners, demonstrate and describe a method for evaluating visual acuity for distant vision.**

3. **On several lab partners, demonstrate and describe a method for evaluating visual acuity for near vision.**

4. **On several lab partners, demonstrate and describe a method for evaluating the direct light reflex.**

5. **On several lab partners, demonstrate and describe performance of the swinging flashlight test.**

6. **In a patient with a lesion involving the left optic nerve, what would you expect to observe in the left eye in response to illumination of the left eye?**

_____

7. **In a patient with a lesion involving the left optic nerve, what would you expect to observe in the right eye in response to illumination of the left eye?**

_____

8. **In a patient with a lesion involving the left optic nerve, what would you expect to observe in the left eye in response to illumination of the right eye?**

_____

9. **In a patient with a lesion involving the left optic nerve, what would you expect to observe in the right eye in response to illumination of the right eye?**

_____

10. In a patient with a lesion involving the right abducens nerve, what would you expect to observe in the left eye in response to illumination of the left eye?

_____

11. In a patient with a lesion involving the right abducens nerve, what would you expect to observe in the right eye in response to illumination of the left eye?

_____

12. In a patient with a lesion involving the right abducens nerve, what would you expect to observe in the left eye in response to illumination of the right eye?

_____

13. In a patient with a lesion involving the right abducens nerve, what would you expect to observe in the right eye in response to illumination of the right eye?

_____

14. In a patient with a lesion involving the right oculomotor nerve, what would you expect to observe in the left eye in response to illumination of the left eye?

_____

15. In a patient with a lesion involving the right oculomotor nerve, what would you expect to observe in the right eye in response to illumination of the left eye?

_____

16. In a patient with a lesion involving the right oculomotor nerve, what would you expect to observe in the left eye in response to illumination of the right eye?

_____

17. In a patient with a lesion involving the right oculomotor nerve, what would you expect to observe in the right eye in response to illumination of the right eye?

_____

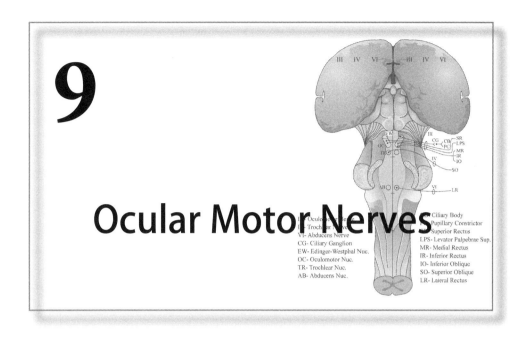

9

Ocular Motor Nerves

III- Oculomotor Nerve
IV- Trochlear Nerve
VI- Abducens Nerve
CG- Ciliary Ganglion
EW- Edinger-Westphal Nuc.
OC- Oculomotor Nuc.
TR- Trochlear Nuc.
AB- Abducens Nuc.

Ciliary Body
Pupillary Constrictor
Superior Rectus
LPS- Levator Palpebrae Sup.
MR- Medial Rectus
IR- Inferior Rectus
IO- Inferior Oblique
SO- Superior Oblique
LR- Lateral Rectus

Neuroscience Review

1. **Define and describe Listing's plane.**

   _____

   _____

2. **Define and describe Fick's axes.**

   a. X axis _____

   _____

   b. Y axis _____

   _____

   c. Z axis _____

   _____

Nolan MF. *Clinical Applications of Human Neuroscience: A Laboratory Guide* (pp 63-69).

3. **List the extraocular muscles and indicate the cranial nerve that innervates each.**

Muscle   **Nerve**

_____   _____

_____   _____

_____   _____

_____   _____

_____   _____

_____   _____

4. **List the primary and secondary actions for each extraocular muscle.**

		Primary Action	**Secondary Actions**	
a.	lateral rectus	_____		
b.	medial rectus	_____		
c.	superior rectus	_____	_____	_____
d.	inferior rectus	_____	_____	_____
e.	superior oblique	_____	_____	_____
f.	inferior oblique	_____	_____	_____

5. **Describe the action for each muscle used for testing that muscle.**

   a. lateral rectus_____

   b. medial rectus _____

   c. superior rectus _____

   d. inferior rectus_____

   e. superior oblique _____

   f. inferior oblique _____

6. **Describe the resting position of the eye in a patient with damage to each of the extra-ocular nerves.**

    a.   abducens nerve_____

    b.   oculomotor nerve_____

    c.   trochlear nerve _____

7. **Where in the brainstem is the oculomotor nucleus located?**

    _____

8. **Where in the brainstem is the trochlear nucleus located?**

    _____

9. **Where in the brainstem is the abducens nucleus located?**

    _____

10. **Which of the ocular motor nerves emerges from the brainstem from its dorsal surface?**

    _____

11. **Which extraocular muscle is innervated by cells located on both the ipsilateral and contralateral sides?**

    _____

12. **Which of the ocular motor nerves passes through (rather than in the wall of) the cavernous sinus?**

    _____

13. **Which of the ocular motor nerves does not pass through the annulus of Zinn?**

    _____

14. **Which of the ocular motor nerves carries autonomic as well as somatic motor fibers?**

    _____

15. According to Sherrington's law, when the right lateral rectus muscle contracts, what other muscle will be affected, and will it contract or relax?

Muscle   **Side**   **Contract/Relax**

_____   _____   _____

16. According to Hering's law, when the right lateral rectus muscle contracts, what other muscle will be affected, and will it contract or relax?

Muscle   **Side**   **Contract/Relax**

_____   _____   _____

17. Where in the brainstem is the center for horizontal gaze?

_____

18. Where in the brainstem is the center for vertical gaze?

_____

19. What is the name of the fiber pathway that interconnects the brainstem gaze centers with the ocular motor nuclei?

_____

20. Which area of the cerebral cortex (Brodmann area) is associated with volitional eye movements and what is the Brodmann number of this area?

Cortical Area   **Brodmann Number**

_____   _____

21. What areas of the cerebral cortex are associated with pursuit (tracking) eye movements and what are the Brodmann numbers of these areas?

Cortical Area   **Brodmann Number**

_____   _____

22. Define the following terms.

a. heterotropia (tropia) _____

_____

b.   comitant heterotropia _____

_____

c.   incomitant heterotropia _____

_____

d.   heterophoria (phoria) _____

_____

e.   strabismus _____

_____

f.   nystagmus _____

_____

g.   diplopia _____

_____

h.   ptosis _____

_____

i.   duction movements _____

_____

j.   version movements _____

_____

k.   vergence movements _____

_____

l.   primary deviation _____

_____

m.   secondary deviation _____

_____

n.   oscillopsia _____

_____

o.   Sherrington's law _____

_____

p.   Hering's law _____

_____

APPLICATION EXERCISES

1. What are the 2 steps involved in the single cover test?

   a. _____

   b. _____

2. What are the 2 steps involved in the cover/uncover test?

   a. _____

   b. _____

3. What are the 2 steps involved in the alternate cover test?

   a. _____

   b. _____

4. On several lab partners, perform and describe a method for evaluating the function of each of the extraocular muscles individually.

5. On several lab partners, perform the single cover test and describe the findings you would expect in a patient with a lesion involving the right abducens nerve.

   _____

6. On several lab partners, perform the cover/uncover test and describe the findings you would expect in a patient with a lesion involving the left abducens nerve.

   _____

7. On several lab partners, perform the alternate cover test and describe the findings you would expect in a patient with an esophoria.

   _____

8. Which of the ocular motor nerves may be injured in a patient with transtentorial (uncal) herniation?

   _____

9. Describe the strabismus expected in a patient with a unilateral lesion involving the right oculomotor nerve.

   _____

10. What movement will result in maximal diplopia in a patient with a lesion that affects the left abducens nerve?

_____

11. Damage to which ocular motor nerve will result in anisocoria?

_____

12. Name the ocular motor abnormality likely to be observed in a patient attempting to look straight ahead who has a lesion affecting the cavernous part of the left carotid artery.

_____

13. If the patient in the above question reports diplopia in the position of primary gaze, shifting the gaze in which direction will result in a worsening of the diplopia?

_____

14. In the patient in the above question, will you expect to find anisocoria? Explain.

_____

_____

_____

15. On several lab partners, demonstrate and describe a method for evaluating volitional eye movements.

16. Describe the findings you would expect in a patient with a destructive lesion involving the posterior part of the frontal lobe on the left side.

_____

_____

17. On several lab partners, demonstrate and describe a method for evaluating pursuit eye movements.

18. Describe the findings you would expect in a patient with a destructive lesion involving the occipital cortex on the left side.

_____

_____

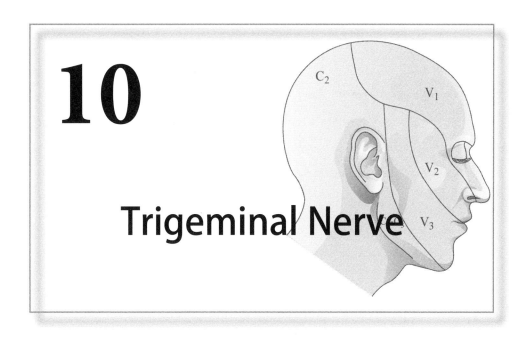

NEUROSCIENCE REVIEW

1. List the 3 divisions of the trigeminal nerve and name the intracranial foramen through which each passes.

	Division	Foramen
a.	_____	_____
b.	_____	_____
c.	_____	_____

2. Name the part of the trigeminal nuclear complex where the nociceptive afferent fibers terminate.

   _____

3. Name the part of the trigeminal nuclear complex where the non-nociceptive afferent fibers terminate.

   _____

Nolan MF. *Clinical Applications of Human Neuroscience:*
A Laboratory Guide (pp 71-75).
© 2014 SLACK Incorporated.

4. Name the tract formed by the trigeminothalamic axons that cross the midline.

   _____

5. Name the tract formed by the trigeminothalamic axons that do not cross the midline.

   _____

6. Name the 3 thalamic nuclei that receive synaptic input from the trigeminothalamic tracts.

   a. _____

   b. _____

   c. _____

7. Name the gyrus where thalamocortical fibers subserving the face terminate.

   _____

8. Which artery supplies the primary sensory cortical area that subserves the face?

   _____

9. Through which limb of the internal capsule do these face-related thalamocortical fibers pass?

   _____

10. Describe the orientation of the homunculus of the face on the primary sensory cortex.

    _____

    _____

    _____

11. Name the nucleus composed of motor neurons with axons that are part of the trigeminal nerve.

    _____

12. Which division of the trigeminal nerve includes these motor axons?

    _____

13. **Name the 4 major muscles innervated by the trigeminal nerve.**

    a. _____

    b. _____

    c. _____

    d. _____

14. **Name the 4 smaller muscles innervated by the trigeminal nerve.**

    a. _____

    b. _____

    c. _____

    d. _____

15. **Name the 4 reflexes in which the trigeminal nerve serves as the afferent limb.**

    a. _____

    b. _____

    c. _____

    d. _____

16. **Name the reflex in which the trigeminal nerve serves as the efferent limb.**

    _____

17. **Where are the nerve cell bodies of the afferent limb of the masseter reflex?**

    _____

18. **In addition to the skin of the face, what 2 other structures or regions of the head receive sensory innervation by way of the trigeminal nerve?**

    a. _____

    b. _____

APPLICATION EXERCISES

1. **On several lab partners, mark and describe the areas of skin innervated by each division of the trigeminal nerve.**

2. On several lab partners, demonstrate and describe a method for evaluating the sensory function of the trigeminal nerve.

3. On several lab partners, demonstrate and describe a method for eliciting the masseter reflex.

4. What is the expected response to elicitation of the masseter reflex in a neurologically intact individual?

_____

5. On several lab partners, demonstrate and describe a method for eliciting the corneal reflex.

6. Indicate the cranial nerves that subserve the afferent limb and the efferent limb of the corneal reflex.

Afferent Limb   **Efferent Limb**

_____   _____

7. What is the expected response to elicitation of the corneal reflex in a neurologically intact individual?

_____

8. On several lab partners, demonstrate and describe a method for evaluating the integrity of the motor division of the trigeminal nerve.

9. Which 2 muscles can be palpated to evaluate the motor division of the trigeminal nerve?

a. _____

b. _____

10. A 40-year-old man presents to the clinic with a sore eye. When you lightly touch the right cornea, both eyes close briskly. When you lightly touch the left cornea, neither eye closes. What structure is affected in this patient and on which side?

Structure Affected   **Side Affected**

_____   _____

11. A 54-year-old woman presents to the clinic with a sore eye. When you lightly touch the right cornea, the right eye closes briskly but the left eye does not close. When you lightly touch the left cornea, the right eye closes briskly but the left eye does not close. What structure is affected in this patient and on which side?

Structure Affected   Side Affected

_____   _____

11

Facial Nerve

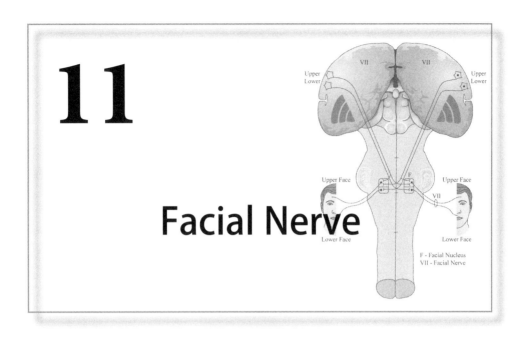

VII VII
Upper Upper
Lower Lower

Upper Face Upper Face
F VII
Lower Face Lower Face

F - Facial Nucleus
VII - Facial Nerve

NEUROSCIENCE REVIEW

1.   List the 2 major divisions of the facial nerve.

   a.   _____

   b.   _____

2.   Name the cranial foramen through which the facial nerves pass to exit the cranial cavity.

   _____

3.   Name the part of the brainstem that marks the attachment of the facial nerve.

   _____

4.   Name the nucleus composed of lower motor nerve cell bodies that is the origin of motor nerve fibers of the facial nerve.

   _____

Nolan MF. *Clinical Applications of Human Neuroscience:*
A Laboratory Guide (pp 77-81).
© 2014 SLACK Incorporated.

5. Name the nucleus composed of nerve cell bodies that are the origin of the auto-
    nomic nerve fibers in the facial nerve.

    _____

6. Name the foramen through which the facial nerve proper passes to exit the skull.

    _____

7. In addition to the muscles of facial expression, list 2 other muscles innervated by the
    facial nerve.

    a. _____

    b. _____

8. Name the 2 parasympathetic ganglia that receive synaptic input from preganglionic
    fibers of the facial nerve.

    a. _____

    b. _____

9. Name the 2 targets of the autonomic nerve fibers of the facial nerve.

    a. _____

    b. _____

10. Name the 2 branches of the facial nerve that carry preganglionic autonomic nerve
    fibers.

    a. _____

    b. _____

11. Name the sensory function of the facial nerve.

    _____

12. Name the ganglion composed of the sensory (afferent) cell bodies of the facial nerve.

    _____

13. Name the nucleus that receives synaptic input from the afferent nerve fibers of the
    facial nerve.

    _____

14. Name the ascending tract (pathway) formed by the axons of the cells of the previously named nucleus.

     _____

15. Name the 2 diencephalic nuclei and 2 brainstem nuclei that receive synaptic input from this ascending gustatory pathway.

     ### Diencephalic Nuclei   ### Brainstem Nuclei

     a. _____   _____

     b. _____   _____

16. Name the gyrus where thalamocortical fibers subserving taste terminate.

     _____

17. Through which limb of the internal capsule do these thalamocortical fibers pass?

     _____

18. Name the gyrus that contains cortical upper motor neurons that innervate the facial nucleus.

     _____

19. Through which limb of the internal capsule do these descending fibers pass?

     _____

20. Define the following terms.

     a. Bell's palsy _____

         _____

     b. Bell's phenomenon _____

         _____

     c. ageusia _____

         _____

APPLICATION EXERCISES

1. Which 4 muscles are commonly tested when evaluating the motor function of the facial nerve?

    a. _____

    b. _____

    c. _____

    d. _____

2. On several lab partners, demonstrate and describe a method for evaluating the somatic motor function of the facial nerve.

3. Which facial muscles will be affected by a lesion that damages the internal capsule on the left side and on which side will each be affected?

    Muscle Affected   **Side Affected**

    _____   _____

    _____   _____

4. Which facial muscles will be affected by a lesion that damages the facial nerve on the right side and on which side will each be affected?

    Muscle Affected   **Side Affected**

    _____   _____

    _____   _____

    _____   _____

    _____   _____

5. A 36-year-old man underwent a surgical procedure in which the chorda tympani was inadvertently damaged on the right side. Which 2 functions will be affected in this patient?

    a. _____

    b. _____

6. A 12-year-old girl was diagnosed with a glioma that has invaded the vidian canal and damaged the neural structure located therein. What sign or symptom would you look for in this girl?

    _____

    _____

7. What symptom would you expect in a patient with a lesion affecting the nerve to the stapedius?

    _____

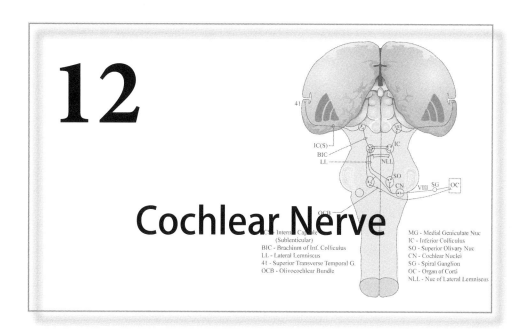

12

Cochlear Nerve

IC(S) - Internal Capsule
(Sublenticular)
BIC - Brachium of Inf. Colliculus
LL - Lateral Lemniscus
41 - Superior Transverse Temporal G.
OCB - Olivocochlear Bundle

MG - Medial Geniculate Nuc
IC - Inferior Colliculus
SO - Superior Olivary Nuc
CN - Cochlear Nuclei
SG - Spiral Ganglion
OC - Organ of Corti
NLL - Nuc of Lateral Lemniscus

NEUROSCIENCE REVIEW

1. Name the middle ear ossicles and indicate the branchial arch from which each is derived.

Ossicle	Branchial Arch
_____	_____
_____	_____
_____	_____

2. Two of the ossicles listed above have muscular attachments. Name the 2 ossicles with attached muscles and name the muscle attached to each.

Ossicle	Muscle
a. _____	_____
b. _____	_____

Nolan MF. *Clinical Applications of Human Neuroscience: A Laboratory Guide* (pp 83-88).
© 2014 SLACK Incorporated.

3. Name the 2 muscles attached to ossicles and name the nerve that innervates each.

    Muscle   **Nerve**

    a. _____   _____

    b. _____   _____

4. On which membrane of the organ of Corti do the auditory receptor cells rest?

    _____

5. Which membrane of the organ of Corti separates the scala vestibuli from the scala media (cochlear duct)?

    _____

6. Which membrane of the organ of Corti separates the scala tympani from the scala media (cochlear duct)?

    _____

7. Which membrane of the organ of Corti makes contact with the cilia of the auditory receptor cells?

    _____

8. Describe the tonotopic organization of the auditory receptor cells. (Which tones are represented at the base and which tones are represented at the apex?)

    a. base _____

    b. apex _____

9. Name the ganglion composed of the afferent cell bodies of the auditory nerve.

    _____

10. Name the cranial foramen through which the auditory nerve passes to enter the cranial cavity.

    _____

11. Name the nuclei where the axons of the auditory nerve terminate.

    _____

    _____

12. Name the 3 decussating pathways that originate from the cochlear nuclei.

    a. _____

    b. _____

    c. _____

13. Which of the above decussating pathways is referred to as the trapezoid body?

    _____

14. Name the ascending auditory pathway that arises from the cochlear nuclei.

    _____

15. Name the nucleus of the midbrain that receives synaptic input from the above-named pathway.

    _____

16. Name the pathway (tract) formed by the axons that arise from the midbrain nucleus named above that terminate in the thalamus.

    _____

17. Name the thalamic nucleus that receives auditory information.

    _____

18. Name the gyrus where thalamocortical fibers subserving auditory function terminate and indicate its Brodmann number.

    ### Gyrus Name   Brodmann Number

    _____   _____

19. Through which limb of the internal capsule do these thalamocortical fibers pass?

    _____

20. Describe the tonotopic organization of the primary auditory cortex. (Which tones are represented anterolaterally and which tones are represented posteromedially?)

    a. anterolateral part _____

    b. posteromedial part _____

21. Which Brodmann areas are referred to as auditory association areas?

_____

22. What specific auditory association area is related to language function?

_____

23. Sudden, loud sounds can elicit 2 reflex responses that help to dampen the movements of the ossicles. List the 2 muscles involved and indicate the nerve that innervates each.

Muscle   **Nerve**

a. _____   _____

b. _____   _____

24. Define the following terms.

a. tonotopia _____

_____

b. hypacusis _____

_____

c. conduction deafness _____

_____

d. sensorineural deafness _____

_____

e. tinnitus _____

_____

f. presbycusis _____

_____

g. stapedius reflex _____

_____

APPLICATION EXERCISES

1. Does most of the auditory information that reaches the cerebral cortex arise from the ipsilateral side or contralateral ear?

   _____

2. On several lab partners, demonstrate and describe a screening method for evaluating auditory function.

3. On several lab partners, demonstrate and describe a method for performing the Rinne test.

4. Which tuning fork is recommended for use when performing the Rinne test?

   _____

5. In a patient with suspected hearing loss in the right ear, the Rinne test reveals that AC > BC. Is this finding suggestive of conduction deafness or sensorineural deafness of the right ear?

   _____

6. In a patient with suspected hearing loss in the left ear, the Rinne test reveals that BC > AC. Is this finding suggestive of conduction deafness or sensorineural deafness of the left ear?

   _____

7. On several lab partners, demonstrate and describe a method for performing the Weber test.

8. Which tuning fork is recommended for use when performing the Weber test?

   _____

9. In a patient with suspected hearing loss in the right ear, the Weber test lateralizes to the left side. Is this finding suggestive of conduction deafness or sensorineural deafness of the right ear?

   _____

10. In a patient with suspected hearing loss in the left ear, the Weber test lateralizes to the left side. Is this finding suggestive of conduction deafness or sensorineural deafness of the left ear?

_____

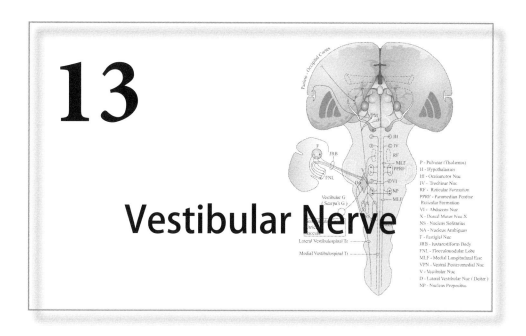

13

Vestibular Nerve

P - Pulvinar (Thalamus)
H - Hypothalamus
III - Oculomotor Nuc
IV - Trochlear Nuc
RF - Reticular Formation
PPRF - Paramedian Pontine
  Reticular Formation
VI - Abducens Nuc
X - Dorsal Motor Nuc X
NS - Nucleus Solitarius
NA - Nucleus Ambiguus
F - Fastigial Nuc
JRB - Juxtarestiform Body
FNL - Flocculonodular Lobe
MLF - Medial Longitudinal Fasc
VPN - Ventral Posteromedial Nuc
V - Vestibular Nuc
D - Lateral Vestibular Nuc (Deiter)
NP - Nucleus Prepositus

Neuroscience Review

1. Which vestibular receptor is responsive to angular (rotatory) acceleration and deceleration and where are these receptors located?

    Receptor   **Location**

    _____   _____

2. Which vestibular receptor is responsive to linear acceleration and deceleration and where are these receptors located?

    Receptor   **Location**

    _____   _____

3. Which of the receptors indicated above is associated with otoconia?

    _____

Nolan MF. *Clinical Applications of Human Neuroscience:*
A Laboratory Guide (pp 89 94).
© 2014 SLACK Incorporated.

4.   Name the ganglion composed of the afferent cell bodies of the vestibular nerve.

_____

5.   Name the cranial foramen through which the vestibular nerve passes to enter the cranial cavity.

_____

6.   Name the nuclei where the axons of the vestibular nerve terminate.

_____

7.   Which of the vestibular nuclei preferentially receive synaptic input from the receptors in the semicircular canals?

_____

8.   Which of the vestibular nuclei preferentially receive synaptic input from the receptors in the utricle and saccule?

_____

9.   Which of the vestibular nuclei preferentially give rise to axons that ascend in the medial longitudinal fasciculus?

_____

10.   Which of the vestibular nuclei preferentially give rise to axons that descend in the medial vestibulospinal tract?

_____

11.   In which region of the spinal cord is the medial vestibulospinal tract located?

_____

12.   Which nucleus gives rise to axons that descend in the lateral vestibulospinal tract?

_____

13.   In which region of the spinal cord is the lateral vestibulospinal tract located?

_____

14.   Which lobe of the cerebellum is reciprocally connected with the vestibular nuclei?

_____

15. What is the name of the fiber pathway that interconnects the vestibular nuclei with the cerebellum?

_____

16. What nucleus of the brainstem receives projections from the vestibular nuclei and plays a role in vomiting?

_____

17. What nucleus of the brainstem receives projections from the vestibular nuclei and plays a role in pharyngeal muscle activity?

_____

18. What region of the brainstem receives projections from the vestibular nuclei and plays a role in mediating sweating and facial pallor?

_____

19. Name 3 nuclei of the diencephalon that receive synaptic input from the vestibular nuclei.

a. _____

b. _____

c. _____

20. What is the effect on impulse frequency in the left vestibular nerve when the head is rotated to the left?

_____

21. Describe the pathophysiological bases for each of the following.

a. vertiginous dizziness _____

_____

b. presyncopal dizziness _____

_____

c. disequilibrium _____

_____

d. lightheadedness _____

_____

22. **Define the following terms.**

a.   vertigo _____

_____

b.   oscillopsia _____

_____

c.   nystagmus _____

_____

d.   positional nystagmus _____

_____

e.   gaze-evoked nystagmus _____

_____

f.   vestibulo-ocular reflexes _____

_____

g.   oculo-vestibular reflex _____

_____

h.   oculo-cephalic reflex _____

_____

i.   canal paresis _____

_____

j.   Dix-Hallpike maneuver _____

_____

k.   Epley maneuver _____

_____

APPLICATION EXERCISES

1.   **Slowly rotate a lab partner to the left on a revolving stool at a rate of 1/2 revolution per second for 8 revolutions. Stop the subject and observe the subject's eyes. Name the type of nystagmus you observe.**

_____

2.   Describe the response you would expect to elicit in a neurologically intact individual in whom you irrigate the right external ear canal with cold water.

_____

3.   Describe a method for eliciting the oculo-cephalic reflex.

_____

_____

_____

4.   Describe a method for eliciting the oculo-vestibular reflex.

_____

_____

_____

5.   Demonstrate the use of past-pointing in the evaluation for suspected vestibular nerve dysfunction.

6.   Describe the observation you might expect when using past-pointing in a patient with damage to the right vestibular nerve.

_____

7.   Demonstrate the use of marching-in-place in the evaluation for suspected vestibular nerve dysfunction.

8.   Describe the observation you might expect when using marching-in-place in a patient with damage to the left vestibular nerve.

_____

9.   Name the type of nystagmus that might be observed in a patient with an acute destructive lesion affecting the right vestibular nerve.

_____

10. Describe the findings you might expect with cold caloric testing of the right side in a patient with a supratentorial lesion.

_____

_____

11. Describe the findings you might expect with cold caloric testing of the right side in a patient with damage to the vestibular nerve on the right side.

    _____

    _____

12. What is the term used to describe the type of rigidity observed in a patient with a lesion above the level of the midbrain?

    _____

13. What is the term used to describe the type of rigidity observed in a patient with a lesion at the level of the mid pons?

    _____

14. A 30-year-old man with dizziness and an imaging-confirmed lesion involving the left vestibular nerve presents to the ear/nose/throat clinic. The patient demonstrates rotation when performing marching-in-place. In which direction will he rotate during this test?

    _____

15. A 42-year-old woman presents with hearing loss and left horizontal jerk nystagmus. She is diagnosed with disease resulting in damage to the vestibular nerve. On which side is her disease?

    _____

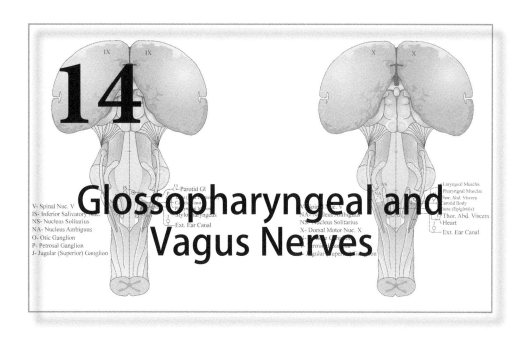

NEUROSCIENCE REVIEW

1. Name the sulcus of the brainstem that marks the attachment of the glossopharyngeal nerve.

   _____

2. Name the cranial foramen through which the glossopharyngeal nerve passes to exit the cranial cavity.

   _____

3. Name the skeletal muscle that is innervated by the glossopharyngeal nerve.

   _____

4. Name the nucleus in the brainstem that is the origin of axons that innervate the muscle indicated above.

   _____

5. Name the gland that is innervated by the glossopharyngeal nerve.

   _____

Nolan MF. *Clinical Applications of Human Neuroscience:*
A Laboratory Guide (pp 95-99).
© 2014 SLACK Incorporated.

6. Name the nucleus in the brainstem that is the origin of preganglionic axons that are part of the glossopharyngeal nerve.

    _____

7. Name the ganglion that receives synaptic input from the preganglionic axons of the glossopharyngeal nerve.

    _____

8. Name the structure that is innervated by the postganglionic nerve cells indicated above.

    _____

9. Name the 2 sensory receptors that, when activated, transmit impulses toward the brainstem by way of the glossopharyngeal nerve and name the sensory ganglia formed by the cell bodies that innervate each.

Receptor	Ganglion
a. _____	_____
b. _____	_____

10. Name the nucleus in the brainstem where the central processes from each of the ganglia listed above terminate.

Ganglion	Brainstem Nucleus
_____	_____
_____	_____

11. Name the sulcus of the brainstem that marks the attachment of the vagus nerve.

    _____

12. Name the cranial foramen through which the vagus nerve passes to exit the cranial cavity.

    _____

13.   Name the skeletal muscle groups that are innervated by the vagus nerve.

_____

_____

14.   Name the muscle innervated by the external laryngeal nerve.

_____

15.   Name the branch of the vagus nerve that innervates the laryngeal muscles.

_____

16.   Name the nucleus in the brainstem that is the origin of axons that innervate the laryngeal muscles.

_____

17.   Name the nucleus in the brainstem that is the origin of axons that influence activity of the heart.

_____

18.   Name the nucleus in the brainstem that is the origin of axons that influence activity of the circular and longitudinal muscles of the small intestine.

_____

19.   Name the ganglion composed of nerve cell bodies with axons that carry afferent (sensory) information from the duodenum.

_____

20.   Name the ganglion composed of nerve cell bodies with axons that carry afferent (sensory) information from the meninges.

_____

21. Name the 2 sensory receptors that, when activated, transmit impulses toward the brainstem by way of the vagus nerve and name the sensory ganglia formed by the cell bodies that innervate each.

Receptor   **Ganglia**

   a. _____   _____

   b. _____   _____

22. Name the nucleus in the brainstem where the afferent (sensory) fibers from the stomach terminate.

_____

23. Name the nucleus in the brainstem where the afferent (sensory) fibers from the meninges terminate.

_____

24. Define the following terms.

   a.   dysarthria _____

_____

   b.   dysphonia _____

_____

   c.   dysphagia _____

_____

APPLICATION EXERCISES

1. Which cranial nerves serve as the afferent and efferent limbs of the pharyngeal (gag) reflex?

Afferent Limb   **Efferent Limb**

_____   _____

2.   Which ganglion is formed in part by the nerve cell bodies of the nerve that serves as the afferent limb of the pharyngeal (gag) reflex?

_____

3.   Which muscle is innervated by the nerve that serves as the efferent limb of the pharyngeal (gag) reflex?

_____

4.   Which muscle forms the posterior pillar of the tonsillar fossa?

_____

5.   Which muscle forms the anterior pillar of the tonsillar fossa?

_____

6.   Which cranial nerve innervates the carotid sinus?

_____

7.   Which cranial nerve innervates the carotid body?

_____

8.   In a patient with a lesion involving the left glossopharyngeal nerve, which way will the uvula deviate when the patient is asked to say "aaahhh"?

_____

9.   In a patient with a lesion involving the right vagus nerve, which way will the uvula deviate when the patient is asked to say "aaahhh"?

_____

10. In a patient with a lesion involving the left glossopharyngeal nerve, what will you likely observe when you touch the right tonsillar fossa?

_____

11. In a patient with a lesion involving the left glossopharyngeal nerve, what will you likely observe when you touch the left tonsillar fossa?

_____

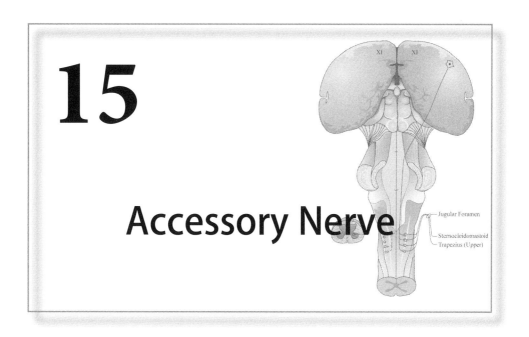

15

Accessory Nerve

Jugular Foramen
Sternocleidomastoid
Trapezius (Upper)

NEUROSCIENCE REVIEW

1. Name the nucleus formed by the cell bodies that give rise to the axons of the accessory nerve.

   _____

2. Are the cortical upper motor neurons that innervate the above-named nucleus located on the ipsilateral or contralateral side?

   _____

3. Name the foramen through which the fibers of the accessory nerve enter the cranial cavity.

   _____

4. Name the foramen through which the fibers of the accessory nerve exit the cranial cavity.

   _____

Nolan MF. *Clinical Applications of Human Neuroscience: A Laboratory Guide* (pp 101-102).
© 2014 SLACK Incorporated.

5.   **Name the 2 muscles innervated by the accessory nerve.**

   a.   _____

   b.   _____

6.   **Define the following term.**

   a.   torticollis _____

   _____

Application Exercise

1.   **On several lab partners, demonstrate and describe a method for evaluating the function of the accessory nerve.**

16

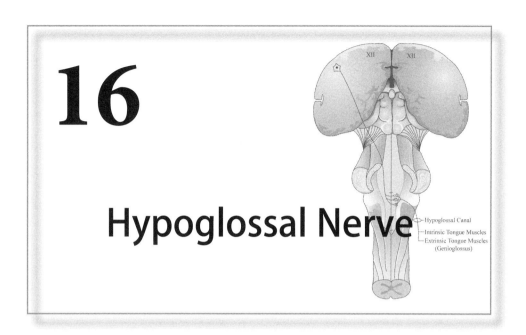

Hypoglossal Nerve

- Hypoglossal Canal
- Intrinsic Tongue Muscles
- Extrinsic Tongue Muscles
  (Genioglossus)

NEUROSCIENCE REVIEW

1. Name the sulcus of the brainstem that marks the attachment of the hypoglossal nerve.

   _____

2. Name the nucleus formed by the cell bodies that give rise to the axons of the hypoglossal nerve.

   _____

3. Are the cortical upper motor neurons that innervate the above-named nucleus located on the ipsilateral or contralateral side?

   _____

4. Name the foramen through which the fibers of the hypoglossal nerve exit the cranial cavity.

   _____

Nolan MF. *Clinical Applications of Human Neuroscience:
A Laboratory Guide* (pp 103-104).
© 2014 SLACK Incorporated.

5. Name the 3 extrinsic muscles of the tongue innervated by the hypoglossal nerve.

    a. _____

    b. _____

    c. _____

6. Name the 1 extrinsic muscle of the tongue that is not innervated by the hypoglossal nerve.

    a. _____

Application Exercises

1. Which extrinsic muscle of the tongue is used to protrude the tongue as part of the evaluation of the hypoglossal nerve?

    _____

2. On several lab partners, demonstrate and describe a method for evaluating the function of the hypoglossal nerve.

3. In a patient with a lesion involving the right hypoglossal nerve, which side of the tongue will demonstrate atrophy?

    _____

4. In a patient with a lesion involving the left hypoglossal nerve, which way will the tongue deviate on protrusion?

    _____

SECTION V

Mental Status

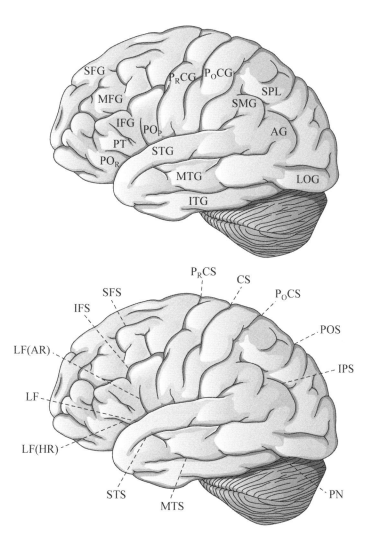

17

Consciousness

NEUROSCIENCE REVIEW

1. **What are the 2 categories of consciousness?**

    a. _____

    b. _____

2. **List 4 terms that refer to altered levels of consciousness.**

    a. _____

    b. _____

    c. _____

    d. _____

3. **List 4 brainstem reflexes commonly used to localize lesions that affect level of consciousness.**

    a. _____

    b. _____

    c. _____

    d. _____

Nolan MF. *Clinical Applications of Human Neuroscience:*
A Laboratory Guide (pp 107-110).
© 2014 SLACK Incorporated.

4. List 4 physiological processes mediated by brainstem centers that may be affected in patients with brainstem lesions that alter level of consciousness.

   a. _____

   b. _____

   c. _____

   d. _____

5. List the 3 categories of responses observed when administering the Glasgow Coma Scale.

   a. _____

   b. _____

   c. _____

6. Decreased level of consciousness suggests brainstem dysfunction. List the main causes of brainstem injury associated with altered level of consciousness.

   a. primary (direct) causes of brainstem injury_____

   _____

   b. secondary (indirect) causes of brainstem injury _____

   _____

7. List 4 cerebral (higher cortical) functions commonly assessed when evaluating a patient with altered content of consciousness.

   a. _____

   b. _____

   c. _____

   d. _____

8. Decreased content of consciousness suggests cerebral dysfunction. List the main cause of cerebral injury associated with altered content of consciousness.

   _____

9. **Describe the alterations in muscle tone and resulting changes in limb position (upper limbs and lower limbs) in a patient who exhibits decerebrate rigidity.**

    a. upper limbs _____

    _____

    b. lower limbs_____

    _____

10. **Describe the alterations in muscle tone and resulting changes in limb position (upper limbs and lower limbs) in a patient who exhibits decorticate rigidity.**

    a. upper limbs _____

    _____

    b. lower limbs_____

    _____

11. **Define the following terms.**

    a. level of consciousness (arousal) _____

    _____

    b. content of consciousness (awareness) _____

    _____

    c. lethargy _____

    _____

    d. obtundation _____

    _____

    e. stupor _____

    _____

    f. coma _____

    _____

    g. confusion _____

    _____

    h. delirium _____

    _____

i. acute confusional state _____

_____

j. vegetative state _____

_____

k. minimally conscious state _____

_____

APPLICATION EXERCISES

1. **On several lab partners, demonstrate and describe a method for evaluating and documenting the results of testing each of the following brainstem reflexes:**

   a. pupillary light reflexes

   b. corneal reflex

   c. vestibulo-ocular reflex (oculo-cephalic reflex)

   d. pharyngeal reflex

2. **On several lab partners, demonstrate and describe a method for evaluating and documenting the results of testing each of the following cerebral functions:**

   a. attention

   b. orientation

   c. memory function

   d. immediate recall

   e. short-term memory

   f. long-term memory

18

Attention

NEUROSCIENCE REVIEW

1. Identify the 3 major nuclei of the ascending reticular activating system and indicate the main neurotransmitter synthesized by the cells that form each.

	Nucleus	Neurotransmitter
a.	_____	_____
b.	_____	_____
c.	_____	_____

2. The axons of the cells identified in the above question ascend to the cerebrum, where they terminate in a wide variety of nuclei and cortical areas. Identify the pathway formed by the axons of these cells as they pass through the diencephalon.

_____

Nolan MF. *Clinical Applications of Human Neuroscience: A Laboratory Guide* (pp 111-112).
© 2014 SLACK Incorporated.

3.   Describe the location within the diencephalon of the pathway identified in the previous question.

_____

4.   Describe the location and function of the reticular nucleus of the thalamus.

_____

_____

5.   Define the following terms.

   a.   reticular formation _____

   _____

   b.   reticular activating system _____

   _____

   c.   delirium _____

   _____

APPLICATION EXERCISES

1.   Demonstrate and describe the method used to evaluate attention embedded in the Mini Mental State Exam.

2.   Demonstrate and describe an alternative and more reliable test for evaluating attention.

_____

19

Orientation

NEUROSCIENCE REVIEW

1. Being oriented indicates an awareness of self and one's surroundings. List the 3 areas of orientation commonly assessed in the neurological exam.

    a. _____

    b. _____

    c. _____

2. List 2 questions that might be asked to evaluate orientation to person.

    a. _____

    b. _____

3. List 5 questions that might be asked to evaluate orientation to place.

    a. _____

    b. _____

    c. _____

    d. _____

    e. _____

Nolan MF. *Clinical Applications of Human Neuroscience: A Laboratory Guide* (pp 113-114). © 2014 SLACK Incorporated.

4.   **List 5 questions that might be asked to evaluate orientation to time.**

   a.   _____

   b.   _____

   c.   _____

   d.   _____

   e.   _____

5.   **Disorientation to which of the previously mentioned is most likely to be indicative of a psychiatric disorder?**

   _____

APPLICATION EXERCISES

1.   **Demonstrate and describe a method for evaluating orientation.**

2.   **Describe a method for documenting the findings in a patient who is disoriented to place.**

20

Language Function

Neuroscience Review

1. Speaking and language are 2 separate functions. Speaking involves the production of sounds. Language involves the use of symbols (auditory or visual) to communicate information. List the 4 physiological operations involved in speaking (speech).

   a. _____

   b. _____

   c. _____

   d. _____

2. What is the term used to describe visual symbols used for communication?

   _____

3. What is the term used to describe auditory symbols used for communication?

   _____

Nolan MF. *Clinical Applications of Human Neuroscience: A Laboratory Guide* (pp 115-119). © 2014 SLACK Incorporated.

4. **Both the left and the right hemispheres are involved in language function. What components of language function are mediated by each?**

Functional Component

a. left hemisphere _____

b. right hemisphere _____

5. **List the 3 major operations associated with oral language function and indicate the main brain regions/structures important for each.**

Language Operation	Important Brain Region/Structure
a. _____	_____
b. _____	_____
c. _____	_____

6. **What are the Brodmann areas (numbers) associated with each of the following?**

a. Broca's area _____

b. Wernicke's area _____

7. **What is the arterial blood supply to Broca's area? (Be specific.)**

_____

8. **What is the arterial blood supply to Wernicke's area? (Be specific.)**

_____

9. **Define the following terms.**

a. fluency _____

_____

b. prosody _____

_____

c. aphasia _____

_____

d. transcortical motor aphasia _____

_____

e. transcortical sensory aphasia _____

_____

f. conduction _____

_____

g. global aphasia _____

_____

h. semantic aphasia _____

_____

i. phonemic aphasia _____

_____

j. neologism _____

_____

k. anomia _____

_____

l. dysphasia _____

_____

m. dysarthria _____

_____

n. dysphonia _____

_____

o. planum temporale _____

_____

APPLICATION EXERCISES

1. **List the 5 language operations commonly evaluated.**

a. _____

b. _____

c. _____

d. _____

e. _____

2. On several lab partners, demonstrate and describe a method for evaluating fluency.

3. On several lab partners, demonstrate and describe a method for evaluating comprehension.

4. On several lab partners, demonstrate and describe a method for evaluating repetition.

5. On several lab partners, demonstrate and describe a method for evaluating object naming.

6. On several lab partners, demonstrate and describe a method for evaluating reading.

7. On several lab partners, demonstrate and describe a method for evaluating writing.

8. What percentage of naturally right-handed individuals who sustain a lesion in the left hemisphere are likely to demonstrate impaired fluency or comprehension?

    _____

9. What percentage of naturally right-handed individuals who sustain a lesion in the right hemisphere are likely to demonstrate impaired fluency or comprehension?

    _____

10. What percentage of naturally left-handed individuals who sustain a lesion in the left hemisphere are likely to demonstrate impaired fluency or comprehension?

    _____

11. What percentage of naturally left-handed individuals who sustain a lesion in the right hemisphere are likely to demonstrate impaired fluency or comprehension?

    _____

12. Describe the clinical findings regarding language function in a right-handed man who sustains a lesion that damages the arcuate fasciculus on the right side.

    _____

    _____

13. What finding on clinical examination helps to distinguish a patient with a Broca's aphasia from a patient with a transcortical motor aphasia?

    _____

14. What finding on clinical examination helps to distinguish a patient with a Wernicke's aphasia from a patient with a transcortical sensory aphasia?

_____

15. Mr. Dextra is a right-handed man with an infarction involving the middle cerebral artery territory in the right cerebral hemisphere. Mr. Sinstra is a left-handed man with an infarction involving the middle cerebral artery territory in the right cerebral hemisphere. Which of these 2 individuals is most likely to demonstrate dysprosody on examination?

_____

16. List the synonyms used to describe Broca's aphasia.

_____

17. List the synonyms used to describe Wernicke's aphasia.

_____

18. What is the most likely location of a lesion that results in a global aphasia?

_____

_____

19. What is the most likely location of a lesion that results in a Broca's aphasia?

_____

_____

20. What is the most likely location of a lesion that results in a Wernicke's aphasia?

_____

_____

21. What is the basic pathophysiological mechanism leading to the development of a transcortical sensory aphasia?

_____

_____

21

Learning and Memory

NEUROSCIENCE REVIEW

1. What is the major cortical area involved in the formation of memories?

   _____

2. What are the 3 cortical structures that compose the hippocampal formation?

   a. _____

   b. _____

   c. _____

3. What is the distinctive histological feature that distinguishes the hippocampal formation from other cortical areas of the hemisphere?

   _____

4. What are the names of the 2 fiber pathways that transmit information into the hippocampal formation from the adjacent cortex (entorhinal cortex)?

   a. _____

   b. _____

Nolan MF. *Clinical Applications of Human Neuroscience:*
A Laboratory Guide (pp 121 124).
© 2014 SLACK Incorporated.

5.   What is Sommer's sector and what is its functional/clinical significance?

    _____

    _____

6.   Where are the cell bodies of fibers referred to as Schaffer collaterals?

    _____

7.   Where are the cell bodies of fibers referred to as mossy fibers?

    _____

8.   What is the location of the majority of cells that give rise to the fornix?

    _____

9.   What 3 nuclei do most of the fibers of the fornix terminate in?

    a.   _____

    b.   _____

    c.   _____

10.   Describe the Papez circuit (beginning in the temporal lobe).

    _____

    _____

    _____

11.   What are the time frames associated with each of the following types of memory?

    a.   working memory _____

    b.   short-term memory _____

    c.   long-term memory_____

12.   Define the following terms.

    a.   hippocampal formation _____

    _____

    b.   hippocampus _____

    _____

c.   cornu ammonis _____

_____

d.   alveus _____

_____

e.   fimbria _____

_____

f.   declarative (explicit) memory _____

_____

g.   procedural (implicit) memory _____

_____

h.   amnesia _____

_____

i.   retrograde _____

_____

j.   anterograde _____

_____

APPLICATION EXERCISES

1.   **List the 4 words that you will use (now and forever more) when you evaluate memory function in your patients. (Hint: Select an object, a color, a characteristic, and a number. Present them to the patient in this order every time.) Write them below, memorize them, and use them consistently.**

a.   (object) _____

b.   (color) _____

c.   (characteristic) _____

d.   (number) _____

2.   **On several lab partners, demonstrate and describe a method for assessing working memory (immediate recall).**

3.   **On several lab partners, demonstrate and describe a method for assessing short-term memory.**

4. On several lab partners, demonstrate and describe a method for assessing long-term memory.

5. In patients who may be unable to speak, visual memory for objects hidden in the room may be tested. On several lab partners, demonstrate a method for evaluating visual memory.

6. Describe a method for documenting findings on memory testing.

   _____

   _____

7. Lesions affecting what cortical area are most likely to result in impaired short-term memory?

   _____

8. Lesions affecting what nuclear structure are most likely to result in impaired short-term memory?

   _____

9. Where are long-term visual memories most likely stored?

   _____

10. Where are long-term auditory memories most likely stored?

   _____

22

Cognitive Function

NEUROSCIENCE REVIEW

Cognitive function (higher cortical function) generally means operations mediated by cells of the cerebral cortex other than simply perceiving stimuli and initiating movement. These functions typically include thinking, planning, judging, deciding, and calculating. The cortical cells involved are described as forming the modality-specific and integrative association cortices of both cerebral hemispheres.

Typical "cognitive functions" tested include fund of knowledge, calculation ability, proverb interpretation, and praxis.

1.   **List the 3 clinical findings that define Balint's syndrome.**

   a.   _____

   b.   _____

   c.   _____

2.   **List the 4 clinical findings that define Gerstmann's syndrome.**

   a.   _____

   b.   _____

   c.   _____

   d.   _____

Nolan MF. *Clinical Applications of Human Neuroscience:*
A Laboratory Guide (pp 125-127).
© 2014 SLACK Incorporated.

3.   Define the following terms.

a.   acalculia _____

_____

b.   gnosia _____

_____

c.   agnosia _____

_____

d.   apperceptive agnosia _____

_____

e.   associative agnosia _____

_____

f.   prosopagnosia _____

_____

g.   stereognosia _____

_____

h.   praxis _____

_____

i.   apraxia _____

_____

j.   ideational apraxia _____

_____

k.   ideomotor apraxia _____

_____

l.   limb-kinetic apraxia _____

_____

m.   buccofacial apraxia _____

_____

n.   dressing apraxia _____

_____

o.   ocular motor apraxia _____

_____

p. constructional apraxia _____

_____

APPLICATION EXERCISES

1. Evaluating fund of knowledge involves having the individual describe/discuss topics of general understanding in areas in which the individual would be expected to have some understanding. An adequate history is required in order to identify appropriate topics for discussion.
    On several lab partners with whom you have some previous familiarity, demonstrate and describe a method for evaluating fund of knowledge. Document your findings as you would in a patient's chart.

2. Calculation ability refers to the ability to correctly perform simple arithmetic calculations and is determined by asking the individual to solve simple arithmetic problems involving addition, subtraction, multiplication, and division.
    On several lab partners, demonstrate and describe a method for evaluating calculation ability. Document your findings as you would in a patient's chart.

3. Proverb interpretation is an example of abstract interpretation. It involves the ability to make an interpretation of a statement other than a literal one.
    On several lab partners, demonstrate and describe a method for evaluating proverb interpretation. Document your findings as you would in a patient's chart.

4. Praxis refers to the ability to perform previously learned movements.
    On several lab partners, demonstrate and describe a method for assessing the ability to perform an intransitive movement.

5. **On several lab partners, demonstrate and describe a method for assessing the ability to perform a transitive movement.**

6. **On several lab partners, demonstrate and describe a method for evaluating tactile gnosis. Document your findings as you would in a patient's chart.**

Answer Key

CHAPTER 1: ANTEROLATERAL SYSTEM

Neuroscience Review

1. high
   slowly

2. mechanical
   chemical
   thermal

3. C   0.5 to 2.0 m/sec
   Aδ   12 to 30 m/sec

4. dorsal horn

5. laminae I, II, V

6. anterior white commissure

7. reticular formation
   superior colliculus

Nolan MF. *Clinical Applications of Human Neuroscience: A Laboratory Guide* (pp 129-165).
© 2014 SLACK Incorporated.

8.   ventral posterolateral (VPL)
     dorsal medial (DM)
     central medial (CM)

9.   postcentral gyrus   upper limb
     posterior paracentral gyrus   lower limb

10. posterior limb

11. cingulate gyrus
     superior frontal gyrus, medial surface

12. anterior limb

13. upper limb—dorsolateral surface
     lower limb—medial surface

14.

Application Exercises

1.

2.

3.

4.

5.

6.

7.

8.   C7 spinal nerve root   left

9.   lateral femoral cutaneous nerve right

10. upper limb   left

11. posterior limb   right

CHAPTER 2: LEMNISCAL SYSTEM

Neuroscience Review

1. low
    rapidly adapting and very rapidly adapting

2. Meissner's corpuscle

3. muscle spindle

4. Aβ   30 to 70 m/sec

5. Ia   70 to 120 m/sec
    II   30 to 70 m/sec

6. dorsal columns

7. fasciculus gracilis   lower limb
    fasciculus cuneatus   upper limb

8. lower limb—medial
    upper limb—lateral

9. nucleus gracilis   lower limb
    nucleus cuneatus   upper limb

10. rostral part of caudal half of medulla oblongata

11. medial lemniscus

12. upper limb—dorsal, lower limb—ventral
    upper limb—medial, lower limb—lateral
    upper limb—ventromedial, lower limb—dorsolateral

13. ventral posterolateral (VPL)

14. upper limb—medial
    lower limb—lateral

15. postcentral gyrus   upper limb
    posterior paracentral gyrus   lower limb

16. posterior limb

17. upper limb—dorsolateral surface
     lower limb—medial surface

18. perception
     localization

19. somatosensory association cortex   interpretation and recognition
     motor and premotor cortex   planning and execution of movements

20.

Application Exercises

1.

2.

3.

4.

5.

6. increased threshold (decreased perception) to stimulation on entire left side of body

7.

8. anesthesia to stimulation on posterior surface of forearm and dorsal surface of hand
    (in distribution of radial nerve)

9. 128 Hz

10.

11. reduced duration of perception

12.

13. increased number of incorrect responses to changes in joint position

14.

15. eyes open—stable
     eyes closed—unstable

16. dorsal columns of spinal cord

17. fasciculus gracilis   right side

18. ventral posterolateral nucleus   right side

19. medial lemniscus   right side

CHAPTER 3: CORTICAL SENSORY FUNCTIONS

Neuroscience Review

1. postcentral gyrus   Brodmann areas 3, 1, 2

2. superior parietal lobule   Brodmann areas 5, 7

3. middle cerebral artery

4. 128 Hz

5. upper limb—index or long finger
    lower limb—great toe

6.

Application Exercises

1.

2. 8 to 10 or until you are satisfied of the reliability of your evaluation

3. 1 to 3 degrees of arc are all that is necessary

4.

5.

6.

7. left side

Chapter 4: Motor Function

Neuroscience Review

1. | *Upper Limb* | *Peripheral Nerve* |
   |---|---|
   | shoulder abduction | **axillary** |
   | elbow flexion | **musculocutaneous** |
   | elbow extension | **radial** |
   | wrist extension | **radial** |
   | wrist flexion | **median** |
   | finger extension | **radial** |
   | finger flexion (grip strength) | **ulnar** |
   | finger abduction | **ulnar** |
   | finger adduction | **ulnar** |

Lower Limb	*Peripheral Nerve*
hip flexion	
hip adduction	**obturator**
hip abduction	**superior gluteal**
hip extension	**inferior gluteal**
knee extension	**femoral**
knee flexion	**sciatic (tibial/common peroneal)**
ankle dorsiflexion	**anterior tibial (deep peroneal)**
ankle plantar flexion	**tibial (posterior tibial)**
toe extension	**anterior tibial (deep peroneal)**

2. | *Upper Limb* | *Spinal Segments* |
   |---|---|
   | shoulder abduction | **C5**, C6 |
   | elbow flexion | C5, **C6** |
   | elbow extension | C7, **C7** |
   | wrist extension | C6, **C7** |
   | wrist flexion | C7, **C8** |
   | finger extension | **C7**, C8 |
   | finger flexion (grip strength) | **C8**, T1 |
   | finger abduction | C8, **T1** |
   | finger adduction | C8, **T1** |

Lower Limb	*Spinal Segments*
hip flexion	L2, L3, **L4**
hip adduction	L2, L3, **L4**
hip abduction	L4, **L5**, S1
hip extension	L5, **S1**, S2
knee extension	L2, L3, **L4**
knee flexion	**L5**, **S1**, S2
ankle dorsiflexion	**L4**, L5
ankle plantar flexion	L5, **S1**, S2
toe extension	L4, **L5**

3. frontal lobe
    parietal lobe

4. upper limbs—frontal
    lower limbs—frontal

5. upper limbs—precentral gyrus
    lower limbs—anterior paracentral gyrus

6. thalamus—posterior limb of the internal capsule
    midbrain—cerebral peduncle
    pons—basis pons (longitudinal pontine bundles)
    medulla oblongata—medullary pyramid

7. pyramidal decussation (decussation of the medullary pyramid)

8. rostral part—upper limb
    caudal part—lower limb

9. 80% to 90%

10. decussate—lateral corticospinal tract
    do not decussate—anterior corticospinal tract

11. upper limb—55%
    lower limb—25%
    non-limb—20%

12. medial part of the ventral horn—axial muscle groups
    intermediate part of the ventral horn—girdle and proximal muscle groups
    lateral part of the ventral horn—distal muscle groups

13. normal (5/5)   full range of motion against gravity with maximal resistance
    good   (4/5)   full range of motion against gravity with some resistance
    fair   (3/5)   full range of motion against gravity only
    poor   (2/5)   full range of motion with gravity eliminated
    trace   (1/5)   palpable or visible muscle contraction with little or no movement
    zero   (0/5)   no palpable or visible muscle contraction

14.

Application Exercises

1.

2. no

3. activity or occupation-related hypertrophy or disuse atrophy

4.

5. ventral horn (lower motor neuron)
   peripheral nervous system (ventral roots, spinal nerve, plexus or peripheral nerves)

6. anterior tibial (deep peroneal) nerve   right side

7. C5 or C6 spinal nerve root   left side

8. ulnar nerve   right side

9. L2 or L3 or L4 spinal nerve root   left side

CHAPTER 5: COORDINATION, STATION, AND GAIT

Neuroscience Review

1. anterior lobe
   posterior lobe
   flocculonodular lobe

2. archicerebellum (vestibulocerebellum)
   paleocerebellum (spinocerebellum)
   neocerebellum (cerebrocerebellum)

3. vermal region
   paravermal region
   hemispheric region

4. primary fissure

5. posterolateral fissure

6. superior cerebellar peduncle   midbrain
    middle cerebellar peduncle   pons
    inferior cerebellar peduncle   medulla oblongata

7. molecular
    Purkinje
    granular

8. stellate
    basket

9. granule
    Golgi

10. *Afferent Tract*   *Efferent Tract*
    superior cerebellar peduncle:
    ventral spinocerebellar tr   cerebello-rubral tr
    trigemino-cerebellar tr   dentato-thalamic tr
                                       cerebello-olivary tr

    middle cerebellar peduncle:
    pontocerebellar tr

    inferior cerebellar peduncle:
    dorsal spinocerebellar tr
    cuneocerebellar tr
    olivo-cerebellar tr

    juxtarestiform body:
    vestibulocerebellar tr   cerebellovestibular tr

11. inferior olivary nucleus

12. nucleus dorsalis (Clarke's nucleus)
    spinal border cells (Stilling's nucleus)

13. vestibular nuclei
    external (accessory, lateral) cuneate nucleus

14. granular layer

15. Purkinje cell

16. gamma aminobutyric acid (GABA)

17. fastigial   vermis
     globose   vermis and paravermal
     emboliform   paravermal
     dentate   hemispheric

18. fastigial   vestibular nuclei
     globose   red nucleus
     emboliform   red nucleus
     dentate   ventral lateral (VL)

19.

Application Exercises

1.

2. upper limb—ataxia with voluntary movement
    lower limb—ataxia (unsteadiness) of gait

3.

4. upper limb—slow, ataxic forearm pronation/supination
    lower limb—slow, ataxic ankle plantar and dorsiflexion

5.

6. standing with eyes open—stable
    standing with eyes closed—unstable

7. dorsal columns of spinal cord

8.

9. heel strike
    foot flat
    heel off
    toe off
    swing phase

10. stiff knee and hip with circumduction during swing phase

11. excessive hip and knee flexion during swing phase with toe hitting before heel

12. unsteady progression, wide-based steps

13. short steps, limited range of motion at all joints, difficulty turning in place

14. dance-like steps, impaired arm swing

15. high stepping with "slapping" of foot at heel strike

16. right side

17. left side

Chapter 6: Muscle Stretch and Cutaneous Reflexes

Neuroscience Review

1. muscle spindle
    Golgi tendon organ

2. muscle spindle

3. muscle elongation (stretch)

4. primary (annulospiral)   Ia
    secondary (flower spray) II

5. Ia   70 to 120 m/sec
    II   30 to 70 m/sec

6. excitation

7. gamma motor neurons   15 to 30 m/sec

8. increase in tension applied to the tendon

9. Ib fiber   70 to 120 m/sec

10. inhibition of lower motor neurons

11. biceps reflex   musculocutaneous
     triceps reflex   radial
     brachioradialis reflex   radial
     finger flexor reflex   median/ulnar
     quadriceps reflex   femoral
     Achilles reflex   tibial (posterior tibial)

12. biceps reflex   <u>C5</u>, C6
     triceps reflex   C6, <u>C7</u>, C8
     brachioradialis reflex   C5, <u>C6</u>, C7
     finger flexor reflex   <u>C8</u>, T1
     quadriceps reflex   L2, L3, <u>L4</u>
     Achilles reflex   L5, <u>S1</u>, S2

13. 0/5   no visible or palpable muscle contraction with reinforcement
     1/5   slight muscle contraction with little or no joint movement
     2/5   distinct muscle contraction with slight joint movement
     3/5   brisk muscle contraction with moderate joint movement
     4/5   strong muscle contraction with 1 to 3 beats of clonus and possible spread
     5/5   strong muscle contraction with sustained clonus

14. *spasticity:*
     velocity dependent
     clasp-knife phenomenon
     more pronounced in antigravity muscles

     rigidity:
     velocity independent
     cog wheeling or lead pipe resistance
     affects all limb muscle groups equally

15. masseter
     Hoffman

16. tactile stimuli (stroking) applied to sole of foot

17. flexion of the toes (downgoing toes)

18. Babinski sign

19. upper motor neuron disease

20.

Application Exercises

1.

2.

3. **threshold**
    latency
    magnitude (amplitude and spread)
    duration

4.

5.

6.

7.

8. **triceps brachii**   **right**

9. **quadriceps femoris**   **left**

10.

11.

CHAPTER 7: OLFACTORY NERVE

Neuroscience Review

1. **olfactory receptor cell**
    Bowman's gland cell
    basal cell
    sustentacular cell

2. **olfactory receptor cell**

3. **pass upward through the cribriform plate of the ethmoid bone**

4. **olfactory bulb**

5.   mitral cells

6.   inhibition

7.   lateral olfactory gyrus (in prepiriform cortex)
     hippocampus
     amygdaloid nucleus

8.   septal nuclei

9.   coffee
     soap
     mint

10. irritant substances activate trigeminal nerve chemoreceptors

11.

Application Exercises

1.

2.

CHAPTER 8: OPTIC NERVE

Neuroscience Review

1.   inversely related both vertically and horizontally

2.   superiorly   60 degrees
     medially   70 degrees
     inferiorly   80 degrees
     laterally   90 degrees

3.   120 degrees (60 degrees in both lateral directions from central vision in primary gaze)

4.   30 degrees (far lateral peripheral vision for each eye—from 60 to 90 degrees from primary gaze)

5. upper nasal   right
    lower nasal   right
    upper temporal   right
    lower temporal   right

6. upper nasal   left
    lower nasal   left
    upper temporal   right
    lower temporal   right

7. posterior

8. 53%

9. lower nasal quadrant of contralateral eye

10. right eye   lower temporal
    left eye   lower nasal

11. right eye   upper nasal
    left eye   upper temporal

12. lateral part

13. lateral part—lingual gyrus
    medial part—cuneate gyrus

14. anterior part—peripheral fields
    occipital pole (posterior part)—central fields (macular fields)

15. posterior cerebral artery

16. Brodmann areas 18 and 19

17. right optic nerve   right anopsia
    left optic tract   right homonymous hemianopsia
    optic chiasm   bitemporal heteronymous hemianopsia
    right lateral geniculate   left homonymous hemianopsia
    left Meyer's loop   right superior homonymous quadrantanopsia

18. far vision

19. near vision

20. Edinger-Westphal nucleus   ciliary ganglion

21. intermediolateral nucleus   superior cervical ganglion

22. optic nerve

23. oculomotor nerve

24. prompt constriction of the pupil in the illuminated eye

25. prompt constriction of the pupil in the nonilluminated eye

26. ocular adduction
    pupillary constriction
    accommodation of the lens

27. right optic nerve

28.

Application Exercises

1.

2.

3.

4.

5.

6. no change in pupil size (no pupillary response)

7. no change in pupil size (no pupillary response)

8. pupillary constriction

9. pupillary constriction

10. pupillary constriction

11. pupillary constriction

12. pupillary constriction

13. pupillary constriction

14. pupillary constriction

15. no change in pupil size (no pupillary response)

16. pupillary constriction

17. no change in pupil size (no pupillary response)

CHAPTER 9: OCULAR MOTOR NERVES

Neuroscience Review

1. a coronal plane that divides the eye into anterior and posterior halves

2. X axis (lateral-horizontal axis)   permits supraduction and subduction
   Y axis (anterior-posterior axis)   permits intorsion and extorsion
   Z axis (vertical axis)   permits abduction and adduction

3. | lateral rectus | abducens |
   |---|---|
   | medial rectus | oculomotor |
   | superior rectus | oculomotor |
   | inferior rectus | oculomotor |
   | superior oblique | trochlear |
   | inferior oblique | oculomotor |

4.
Muscle	Primary Action	Secondary Actions	
lateral rectus	abduction		
medial rectus	adduction		
superior rectus	supraduction	adduction	intorsion
inferior rectus	subduction	adduction	extorsion
superior oblique	intorsion	subduction	abduction
inferior oblique	extorsion	supraduction	abduction

5.   lateral rectus   abduction
         medial rectus   adduction
         superior rectus   supraduct the abducted eye
         inferior rectus   subduct the abducted eye
         superior oblique   subduct the adducted eye
         inferior oblique   supraduct the adducted eye

6.   abducens nerve   adducted
         oculomotor nerve   subducted and abducted
         trochlear nerve   extorted and supraducted

7.   rostral midbrain

8.   caudal midbrain

9.   caudal pons

10.   trochlear nerve

11.   levator palpebrae superioris

12.   abducens nerve

13.   trochlear nerve

14.   oculomotor nerve

15.   medial rectus   right side   relax

16.   medial rectus   left side   contract

17.   paramedian pontine reticular formation (PPRF)

18.   rostral interstitial nucleus of the medial longitudinal fasciculus (riMLF)

19.   medial longitudinal fasciculus (MLF)

20.   prefrontal eye fields   area 8

21.   visual association cortex   areas 18 and 19

22.

Application Exercises

1. cover fixating eye
    observe response of nonfixating eye

2. cover an eye
    uncover the eye and observe the response in that eye

3. alternately cover each eye
    observe the response in the uncovered eye

4.

5. cover the fixating left eye
    observe abduction in the nonfixating right eye to take up fixation

6. cover the right eye
    uncover the right eye and observe abduction of the right eye to take up fixation
    	or
    cover the left eye
    uncover the left eye and observe that it remains adducted

7. the alternately uncovered eye will abduct to take up fixation

8. oculomotor nerve

9. exotropia and subduction of the right eye

10. left lateral gaze shift

11. oculomotor nerve

12. esotropia involving the left eye

13. to the left

14. no—abducens nerve does not innervate pupillary muscles

15.

16. impaired gaze shift to the right

17.

18. impaired visual pursuit from primary gaze to the left

Chapter 10: Trigeminal Nerve

Neuroscience Review

1. ophthalmic   superior orbital fissure
    maxillary   foramen rotundum
    mandibular   foramen ovale

2. spinal trigeminal nucleus (pars caudalis)

3. principal (main, chief sensory) trigeminal nucleus

4. ventral trigeminothalamic tract

5. dorsal trigeminothalamic tract

6. ventral posteromedial nucleus (VPM)
    dorsal medial nucleus (DM)
    central medial nucleus (CM)

7. postcentral gyrus

8. middle cerebral artery

9. posterior limb

10. forehead and scalp—dorsal
    mid face—intermediate
    chin and mouth—ventral

11. masticator (motor) nucleus

12. mandibular

13. masseter
    temporalis
    lateral pterygoid
    medial pterygoid

14. tensor tympani
anterior belly of digastric
mylohyoid
tensor veli palatini

15. corneal reflex
lacrimal reflex
sneeze reflex
masseter reflex

16. masseter reflex

17. mesencephalic nucleus

18. meninges
anterior part of oral cavity, including tongue, teeth, and gingiva

Application Exercises

1.

2.

3.

4. no contraction of the masseter muscle

5.

6. ophthalmic nerve (V1)   facial nerve (VII)

7. bilateral contraction of the orbicularis oculi

8.

9. masseter muscle
temporalis muscle

10. trigeminal nerve   left

11. facial nerve   left

CHAPTER 11: FACIAL NERVE

Neuroscience Review

1. facial nerve proper
   nervous intermedius

2. internal auditory meatus

3. pontomedullary angle

4. facial nucleus

5. superior salivatory nucleus

6. stylomastoid foramen

7. stapedius
   posterior belly of the digastric

8. pterygopalatine ganglion
   submandibular ganglion

9. lacrimal gland
   salivary glands (submandibular and sublingual glands)

10. greater superficial petrosal nerve
    chorda tympani

11. taste appreciation from the anterior two-thirds of the tongue

12. geniculate ganglion

13. nucleus solitarius

14. solitariothalamic tract

15. ventral posteromedial   nucleus ambiguus, reticular formation
    hypothalamus   hypoglossal nucleus, dorsal motor nucleus

16. postcentral gyrus or insula

17. posterior limb of the internal capsule

18. precental gyrus

19. genu of the internal capsule

20.

Application Exercises

1. frontalis
    orbicularis oculi
    risorius
    orbicularis oris

2.

3. risorius   right
    orbicularis oris   right

4. frontalis   right
    orbicularis oculi   right
    risorius   right
    orbicularis oris   right

5. taste perception
    salivation

6. dry, possibly sore eye on ipsilateral side

7. hyperacusis

CHAPTER 12: COCHLEAR NERVE

Neuroscience Review

1. malleus   1st
    incus   1st
    stapes   2nd

2. malleus   tensor tympani
    stapes   stapedius

3. tensor tympani   trigeminal
    stapedius   facial

4. basilar membrane

5. Reissner's membrane

6. basilar membrane

7. tectorial membrane

8. high frequency at base
   low frequency at apex

9. spiral (cochlear) ganglion

10. internal auditory meatus

11. dorsal and ventral cochlear nuclei

12. dorsal acoustic stria
    intermediate acoustic stria
    ventral acoustic stria (trapezoid body)

13. ventral acoustic stria

14. lateral lemniscus

15. nucleus of the inferior colliculus

16. brachium of the inferior colliculus

17. medial geniculate nucleus

18. superior transverse temporal gyrus   area 41

19. sublenticular part of posterior limb of internal capsule

20. anterolateral—low frequency
    posteromedial—high frequency

21. 42 and 22

22. Wernicke's area

23. tensor tympani   trigeminal nerve
    stapedius   facial nerve

24.

Application Exercises

1. contralateral ear

2.

3.

4. 512 Hz

5. sensorineural deafness

6. conduction deafness

7.

8. 512 Hz

9. sensorineural deafness

10. conduction deafness

CHAPTER 13: VESTIBULAR NERVE

Neuroscience Review

1. crista ampullaris   semicircular canals

2. macula   utricle and saccule

3. macula

4. vestibular (Scarpa's) ganglion

5. internal auditory meatus

6.   superior, medial, lateral, and inferior vestibular nuclei

7.   superior and medial

8.   inferior and lateral

9.   superior and medial

10.   medial

11.   anterior funiculus

12.   lateral vestibular nucleus

13.   ventrolateral fasciculus

14.   flocculonodular lobe

15.   juxtarestiform body

16.   dorsal motor nucleus (of X)

17.   nucleus ambiguus

18.   reticular formation

19.   ventral posteromedial (VPM)
      hypothalamus
      pulvinar

20.   impulse frequency increases

21.

22.

Application Exercises

1.   right horizontal nystagmus

2.   left horizontal nystagmus

3. with subject supine, rotate head slowly from side to side and observe eyes

4. with subject supine and head flexed 30 degrees, irrigate one ear with cold water and observe eyes

5.

6. past-pointing to the right side

7.

8. marching-in-place with rotation to the left

9. left horizontal nystagmus

10. tonic deviation of the eyes to the right

11. no ocular response

12. decorticate rigidity

13. decerebrate rigidity

14. to the left

15. right side

CHAPTER 14: GLOSSOPHARYNGEAL AND VAGUS NERVES

Neuroscience Review

1. postolivary sulcus

2. jugular foramen

3. stylopharyngeus

4. nucleus ambiguus

5. parotid gland

6. inferior salivatory nucleus

7. otic ganglion

8. parotid gland

9. carotid sinus   petrosal (inferior) ganglion
   mechanoreceptor   jugular (superior) ganglion

10. petrosal (inferior) ganglion   nucleus solitarius
    jugular (superior) ganglion   spinal trigeminal nucleus

11. postolivary sulcus

12. jugular foramen

13. pharyngeal muscles
    laryngeal muscles

14. cricothyroid muscle

15. inferior branch of recurrent laryngeal nerve

16. nucleus ambiguus

17. dorsal motor nucleus

18. dorsal motor nucleus

19. nodose (inferior) ganglion

20. jugular (superior) ganglion

21. carotid body   nodose
    mechanoreceptor   jugular

22. nucleus solitarius

23. spinal trigeminal nucleus

24.

Application Exercises

1. glossopharyngeal nerve   vagus nerve

2. petrosal ganglion

3. levator veli palatini (superior pharyngeal constrictor)

4. palatopharyngeus

5. palatoglossus

6. glossopharyngeal nerve

7. vagus nerve

8. straight up in the midline

9. to the left

10. bilateral pharyngeal muscle contraction (normal response)

11. no pharyngeal muscle contraction (no response)

CHAPTER 15: ACCESSORY NERVE

Neuroscience Review

1. accessory nucleus

2. ipsilateral side

3. foramen magnum

4. jugular foramen

5. sternocleidomastoid
    trapezius

6.

Application Exercise

1.

CHAPTER 16: HYPOGLOSSAL NERVE

Neuroscience Review

1. **preolivary sulcus**

2. **hypoglossal nucleus**

3. **contralateral side**

4. **hypoglossal canal**

5. **styloglossus**
    hyoglossus
    genioglossus

6. **palatoglossus**

Application Exercises

1. **genioglossus**

2.

3. **right side**

4. **to the left**

CHAPTER 17: CONSCIOUSNESS

Neuroscience Review

1. **level of consciousness (arousal)**
    content of consciousness (awareness)

2. lethargy
    obtundation
    stupor
    coma

3. pupillary light reflexes
    corneal reflex
    pharyngeal (gag) reflex
    vestibulo-ocular reflexes

4. blood pressure
    heart rate
    respiration rate
    sweating (galvanic skin response)

5. eye opening
    best verbal response
    best motor response

6. primary—trauma and vascular
    secondary—compression/displacement

7. attention
    orientation
    cognitive function
    memory

8. toxic/metabolic

9. upper limbs—increased tone and extension
    lower limbs—increased tone and extension

10. upper limbs—increased tone and flexion
    lower limbs—increased tone and extension

11.

Application Exercises

1.

2.

CHAPTER 18: ATTENTION

Neuroscience Review

1.   locus coeruleus   norepinephrine
    raphe nuclei   serotonin
    ventral tegmental area   dopamine

2.   medial forebrain bundle

3.   lateral hypothalamus

4.   between the internal capsule and the thalamic external medullary lamina
    modulates (inhibits) thalamocortical activity

5.

Application Exercises

1.

2.   list (recite) the months of the year forward, then backward

CHAPTER 19: ORIENTATION

Neuroscience Review

1.   person
    place
    time
    (situation)

2.   what is your name?
    who am I?

3.   what country are we in?
    what state are we in?
    what county are we in?
    what city are we in?
    what kind of a place are we in?

4.   what year is this?
     what season is this?
     what month is this?
     what day of the week is this?
     what is the date today?

5.   person

Application Exercises

1.

2.

Chapter 20: Language Function

Neuroscience Review

1.   respiration
     phonation
     resonation
     articulation

2.   graphemes

3.   phonemes

4.   left hemisphere—propositional components
     right hemisphere—prosodic components

5.   fluency   Broca's area
     comprehension   Wernicke's area
     repetition   arcuate fasciculus

6.   Broca's area   44, 45
     Wernicke's area   42, 22

7.   superior branch of the middle cerebral artery

8.   inferior branch of the middle cerebral artery

9.

Application Exercises

1. fluency
    comprehension
    repetition
    reading
    writing

2.

3.

4.

5.

6.

7.

8. 95%

9. 5%

10. 70%

11. 30%

12. impaired repetition with relatively preserved fluency and comprehension

13. repetition is relatively intact

14. repetition is relatively intact

15. Mr. Dextra

16. nonfluent, expressive, motor, anterior

17. fluent, receptive, sensory, posterior

18. proximal (main stem) segment of the middle cerebral artery (M1 segment) on the left side

19. superior branch of the middle cerebral artery on the left side

20. inferior branch of the middle cerebral artery on the left side

21. heart (pump) failure/hypovolemia/hypoperfusion

CHAPTER 21: LEARNING AND MEMORY

Neuroscience Review

1. hippocampal formation of the medial temporal lobe

2. dentate gyrus
   hippocampus (cornu ammonis)
   subiculum

3. it is 3 layered (archicortex)

4. perforant pathway
   alveolar pathway

5. CA1 region of the hippocampus—high susceptibility to hypoxia

6. CA3 region of the hippocampus

7. dentate gyrus

8. subiculum

9. mammillary nuclei
   anterior nucleus of the thalamus
   septal nuclei (area)

10. temporal lobe → mammillary nucleus → anterior thalamic nucleus → cinguate ctx → temporal lobe

11. working memory—seconds
    short-term memory—minutes to days
    long-term memory—months to years

12.

Application Exercises

1.

2.

3.

4.

5.

6. the description should include statements about the integrity of immediate recall, short-term memory, and long-term memory

7. hippocampal formation in medial temporal lobe

8. mammillary nuclei

9. occipital association cortices

10. temporal association cortices

CHAPTER 22: COGNITIVE FUNCTION

Neuroscience Review

1. simultagnosia
    ocular apraxia
    optic ataxia

2. agraphia
    acalculia
    finger agnosia
    right/left confusion

3.

Application Exercises

1.

2.

3.

4.

5.

6.

Index